Foot and Ankle Disorders - Pathology and Surgery

Edited by Dimitrios D. Nikolopoulos and George K. Safos

Published in London, United Kingdom

Foot and Ankle Disorders - Pathology and Surgery
http://dx.doi.org/10.5772/intechopen.105334
Edited by Dimitrios D. Nikolopoulos and George K. Safos

Contributors
Divyashri Nazare, Nicole Marie Smith, H. John John Visser, Chandrasekaran Kuppusamy, Senthil Selvam Pannir Selvam, Sandhiya Manohar, Madhumathi Kuppuraj, Sharmila Subramani, Karthikeyan Shanmugam, Jayaseelan Vijayalakshmi Kunaseelan, Manjula Subramanian, Andrej Čretnik, Elif Tuğçe Çil, Dimitrios D. Nikolopoulos

First published in London, United Kingdom, 2023 by IntechOpen
IntechOpen is the global imprint of INTECHOPEN LIMITED, registered in England and Wales, registration number: 11086078, 5 Princes Gate Court, London, SW7 2QJ, United Kingdom

British Library Cataloguing-in-Publication Data
A catalogue record for this book is available from the British Library

Additional hard and PDF copies can be obtained from orders@intechopen.com

Foot and Ankle Disorders - Pathology and Surgery
Edited by Dimitrios D. Nikolopoulos and George K. Safos
p. cm.
Print ISBN 978-1-83768-907-1
Online ISBN 978-1-83768-908-8
eBook (PDF) ISBN 978-1-83768-909-5

For EU product safety concerns:
IN TECH d.o.o., Prolaz Marije Krucifikse Kozulić 3, 51000 Rijeka, Croatia,
info@intechopen.com or visit our website at intechopen.com.

Meet the editors

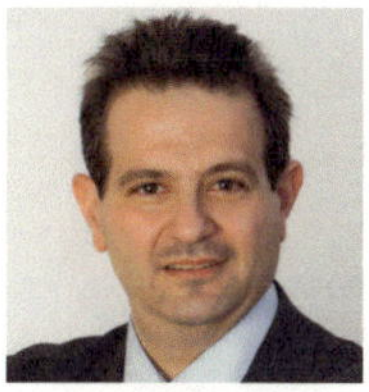

Dr. Dimitrios D. Nikolopoulos is a graduate of Athens University Medical School. He specialized in Orthopaedic Surgery and Traumatology in one of the best clinics in Greece, the Orthopaedic Clinic of the General Hospital "ASKLEPEION" Voulas, where he focused on sports injuries and foot pathology. He continued with a specialization in the pathology of hands in the Microsurgery Clinic of "KAT" Hospital. He proceeded to train alongside Dr. Alexis Nogier at the Clinic Maussins-Nollet in Paris with Arthroscopic Restoration of Hip Pathology and has continued his training in arthroscopic rehabilitation of Sports Injuries of Knee, Shoulder and Ankle, as well as the treatment and surgical correction of foot disorders. He has published 42 original scientific articles in prestigious scientific journals in the USA, Europe and Greece referring to knee surgery (valgus knee) and shoulder (arthroscopic and minimally invasive new techniques), osteoporotic spine and hip fractures, research in vitro environment on bone and cartilage metabolism. He counts over 220 citations in research projects. He has also presented over 180 oral and poster presentations internationally within the last decade namely on sports injury of knee, shoulder, ankle joints and arthritis of the knee and hip. He is a Doctor of the University of Athens and a member of the Greek Traumatology and Orthopaedic Society, the Greek Arthroscopy Society, the European Arthroscopy Association ESSKA and ESSKA_AFAS, as well as other internationally accredited associations.

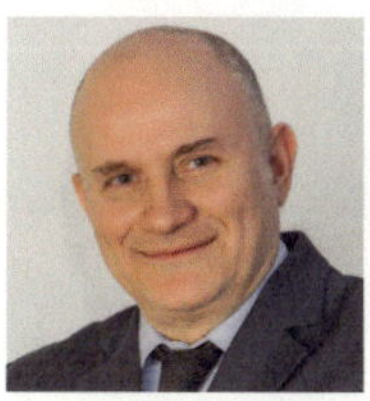

Dr. George K. Safos (MD) specializes in orthopaedic surgery and traumatology with an interest in sports medicine (knee, hip, ankle, elbow, and shoulder arthroscopic surgery) as well as total hip and knee replacement surgery. As a well-published doctor, he now serves as a medical orthopaedic consultant and the primary doctor to various athletic teams, dance groups as well as foreign diplomatic missions. He is a graduate of Athens University Medical School and completed his residency in Orthopaedic Surgery and Traumatology at the General Hospital of Asklepeion Voulas. He then completed two fellowships in the USA, namely at the National Institutes of Health (NIH) in Bethesda, Maryland as well as at The University of Miami-Orthopaedic Department. A post-graduate degree in Tissue Banking at The National University of Singapore with a United Nations scholarship soon followed.

Contents

Preface **IX**

Section 1
Introduction **1**

Chapter 1 **3**
Introductory Chapter: Foot and Ankle Disorders – Pathology and Surgery
by Dimitrios D. Nikolopoulos

Section 2
Arthropathies **9**

Chapter 2 **11**
Ankle-Foot Arthropathies
by Divyashri Nazare

Section 3
Forefoot Pathologies **33**

Chapter 3 **35**
Perspective Chapter: Podological Deformities and Its Management
by Chandrasekaran Kuppusamy, Senthil Selvam Pannir Selvam, Sandhiya Manohar, Madhumathi Kuppuraj, Sharmila Subramani, Karthikeyan Shanmugam, Jayaseelan Vijayalakshmi Kunaseelan and Manjula Subramanian

Chapter 4 **55**
Reconstruction of the Supple Flatfoot with the Concept of Planal Dominance
by H. John Visser and Nicole Marie Smith

Section 4
Causes and Effects of Hindfoot **77**

Chapter 5 **79**
Hindfoot Pathologies
by Elif Tuğçe Çil

Section 5
Achille Tendon Rupture **97**

Chapter 6 **99**
Functional Rehabilitation after Achilles Tendon Rupture
by Andrej Čretnik

Preface

Foot and ankle pathology and disorders have been augmented in the last two decades due to the way of life of the current human beings. On the one hand, the trauma categories are because of motorbike and car accidents; and on the other hand, the chronic syndromes are due to everyday overuse of foot and ankle, as in high-demand sports and hobbies. This book offers an updated guide to foot and ankle pathology, and presents everyday trauma categories, as also chondral and joint chronic syndromes at different ages, which will allow the reader to analyze and understand how the foot develops from the early stages to adulthood.

This book offers an updated guide to the foot and ankle and presents the most common pathology, the conservative therapies and the open or arthroscopic techniques performed worldwide. It provides a general overview of the anatomy, biomechanics, diagnosis, surgical approaches, treatment alternatives, and complications in connection with sports medicine and adult foot and ankle problems, gathering in-depth information on frequent pathologies in a single source. The text is concise and informative, providing a general overview of each disorder, identifying key points for correct diagnosis and differential diagnosis, and highlighting tips and pitfalls in conservative and operative treatment. Written by world-renowned experts in Orthopaedic Surgery, the book offers various points of view on the topics discussed. This comparative approach is generally lacking in foot and ankle literature, an oversight that the book addresses. The content consists of different chapters, divided into the following major sections: "Introduction", "Arthropathies", "Forefoot Pathologies", "Causes and Effects of Hindfoot " and "Achille Tendon Rupture".

Dr. Dimitrios D. Nikolopoulos and Dr. George K. Safos (MD)
Orthopaedic Surgeon, Arthroscopist
Central Clinic of Athens, Greece

Section 1

Introduction

Chapter 1

Introductory Chapter: Foot and Ankle Disorders – Pathology and Surgery

Dimitrios D. Nikolopoulos

1. Introduction

The number of cases of "Foot and ankle Pathology & Disorders" has been augmented in the last two decades due to the current way of life of the human beings. On the one hand are the trauma categories because of motorbike and car accidents; and on the other hand are the chronic syndromes due to everyday overuse of foot and ankle, as in high demand sports and hobbies, as also in ballet dancing, etc.

This book offers an updated guide to the foot and ankle pathology, and presents everyday trauma categories, as also chondral and joint chronic syndromes at all ages from childhood to adults. Furthermore, the book will allow the reader to evaluate and realize how the foot changes during development from the early stages to adulthood. It also provides an overall outline of the anatomy and foot biomechanics, as also diagnosis of the pathologies, the open or arthroscopic surgical approaches, the treatment alternatives, and complications.

Our book, written by world-renowned experts, offers various points of view on the topics discussed, mainly in six chapters, divided into the following sections: (1) Anatomy and biomechanics of foot and ankle, (2) Basic foot and ankle arthropathies, (3) Hindfoot pathologies, (4) Pediatric orthopedics and flatfoot reconstruction, (5) Podological deformities and management, and (6) Achilles tendon rupture and functional rehabilitation.

"Foot and Ankle Disorders - Pathology and Surgery" will be of major interest for orthopedic residents, as also for orthopedic surgeons at the first steps of their career, and for experienced surgeons seeking updated information.

2. Foot and ankle: anatomy and biomechanics

The foot and ankle are a complex of joints made up of 26 individual bones of the foot. The ankle joint—due to the presence of the structure called ankle mortise—provides a high stability role. The ankle complex motions are dorsiflexion 20 degrees, plantarflexion 55 degrees in the sagittal plane; and inversion 30 degrees with eversion 20 degrees in the frontal plane. When these motions occur as coupled motions, they produce the known supination and pronation movements. The range of motion that is available for dorsiflexion will be around 10–20 degrees and for plantar flexion it will be around 40–55 degrees. The forces acting on the ankle joint bear approximately five times the body weight during stance in a normal walking phase and up to 13 times the body weight during running activities [1, 2].

During the daily living activity, the ankle joint possesses high congruency, because first it has a high stability role and second the load-bearing area is larger and mostly in the stance phase during normal gait. The maximum power of the ankle complex is generated around 50% in gait cycle during the forefoot rocker phase correspondingly with the force production of the plantar flexors which is required for the lower extremity to propel the body forward toward toe-off. The other form of stability for foot is provided by the presence of plantar aponeurosis, which takes up to 60% of the weight bearing and the action tie beam around 25% from the metatarsals. The toe extension during the normal gait cycle makes the plantar aponeurosis to become taut, thereby increasing the ability to withstand larger amount of stress [1, 3].

3. Ankle foot arthropathies

In this chapter, the basic pathologies of foot and ankle are analyzed. To be more specific, in the first part of the chapter, the trauma issues of the ankle, such as ankle sprain, calcaneus or talus fractures, and ankle instability, are presented. In the second part of the chapter, the inflammatory conditions, such as osteoarthritis of foot and ankle, rheumatoid arthritis, gouty arthritis, or neuropathic arthritis, are analyzed. In the third part of the chapter, the congenital foot deformities, such as Club foot or Rocker bottom flat foot and other acquired pathologies as Pes planus and cavus, Hallux valgus, Morton's or Hammer toe, are described [4–7].

One of the main problems in 14–17% of patients after ankle sprain pertains to the Osteochondral Lesions (OCLs) of the Talus and these lesions are presented with intermittent or deep pain of the ankle, swelling, plus locking and catching, thereby limiting the patients' mobility. And although it is widely accepted that the small talus OCLs may be treated nonoperatively, the question that easily arises is which is the best surgical technique for these patients with large OCLs. Traditionally, the treatment of small symptomatic OCLs includes either bone marrow stimulation usually with arthroscopic procedures or autologous osteochondral transplantation. Nevertheless, in adults with large OCLs of the talus (>200 mm^2) (focal and contained), the treatment can be challenging, as, on the one hand, the injured articular cartilage shows poor intrinsic reparative competence and, on the other hand, the prescribed techniques till nowadays cannot always offer high success rates in a long-lasting follow-up [7]. In the last decade, taking into consideration first that the periosteum has intrinsic regenerative and regrowth cartilage characteristics; and second that the fresh bone autograft and the aspirated bone marrow contain live mesenchymal precursor cells, novel and innovative technique for ankle OCLs has been presented [8].

4. Hindfoot pathologies

Pain in the foot is prevalent throughout the population, with an estimated range from 17 to 30%. Moreover, more than 25% of the population over the age of 45 have everyday hindfoot pain, which limits their daily activities, causes poor balance and important gait issues, and offers poor health-related quality of life. According to recent studies, at least two-thirds of people have moderate functional daily living issues. Different risk factors for hindfoot pain and pathologies have been identified and analyzed in the literature, such as age, female gender, obesity, posttraumatic osteoarthritis, diabetes, biomechanical factors (lower extremity excessive external rotation, significant pronation of the subtalar joint, weakness of the plantar flexor, and shortening of the achilles tendon), and anatomical variations (pes planus and pes cavus). In this chapter, an overview of the pathologies of the hindfoot that cause hindfoot pain, mainly in patients with bone and soft-tissue overload, foot anatomic disorders, and a decreased range of motion, is provided.

Hindfoot pathologies can be caused by a variety of factors, including overuse, trauma, degeneration, and underlying medical conditions [9, 10]. Some common hindfoot pathologies include tendinopathy of the posterior tibialis tendon or flexor hallucis longus, posterior ankle impingement syndrome (PAIS), calcaneus contusion, stress fractures of the calcaneus or talus, hindfoot rheumatoid arthritis, Paget's disease, osteomyelitis after posterior foot and ankle open fractures, and cancer metastases [9, 10]. One of the most common problems of hindfoot pathology (mainly in athletes and ballet dancers) is the Posterior Ankle Impingement Syndrome (PAIS), which is usually caused by Os Trigonum (OT) or a hypertrophic posterior talar process Stieda. The most common accessory bone of the foot—although usually asymptomatic, it is true that it may become a severely debilitating problem not only for recreational or competitive athletes, but also for ordinary people in their everyday living. Ankles' posterior arthroscopy (PA) has been improved considerably in the last 25 years and has become the gold standard procedure for different pathologies of the ankle and hindfoot, as a safe and reliable treatment option. Currently, the indications for ankles' posterior endoscopy have extended, including both intra- and extra-articular pathologies, and may involve: (1) bone (os trigonum (OT), loose bodies, posttraumatic ossifications, lateral or medial malleolus avulsion fragments, and Haglund's pathology); (2) cartilage (ankle and subtalar joint osteochondral defects, osteoarthritis, osteochondromatosis, and cystic lesions); or (3) soft tissues (tendinopathy of flexor hallucis longus, inflammation of retrocalcaneal bursa, posttraumatic synovitis, and soft-tissue impingement) [9, 10].

Apart from the OT fractures, the further conditions of posterior impingement should be initially treated conservatively (rest, nonsteroidal anti-inflammatory drugs (NSAIDs), and physiotherapy); but when these measures fail, or if we are dealing with high-performance athletes—surgical treatment should be considered early. Of course, it is particularly important for the orthopedic surgeon to assess preoperatively to which of these three categories the patient belongs, so as to be accurate in treating the exact problem [9, 10]. Hence, the purpose of the present chapter is to evaluate the efficiency and the effectiveness of surgical and conservative techniques in hindfoot pathologies; and also, to assess the level of function, outcome measures, and physical examination parameters, with the purpose of providing the readers an overview of clinical results after performing an open or arthroscopic operation. This chapter will help the orthopedic surgeons to manage their patients' expectations after arthroscopy. It is well known that arthroscopic techniques offer earlier recovery with limited pain, significant improvement in the joint function, and restoration of ankle motion with limited complications versus the open techniques.

5. Flatfoot reconstruction

One of the most common presenting problems in orthopedic surgeons' everyday practice is the painful flatfoot. The flatfoot pathologies are treated first conservatively with customized orthotics to support the counter arch, and shoe alterations and second with physiotherapy, providing excellent outcomes (heel cord stretching exercises, foot strengthening of the dorsiflexors and invertors). Nevertheless, in some cases, conservative care may not alleviate the associated symptoms of lower limb or the lumbar spine [11, 12].

Management of the adolescent and flexible flatfoot deformity represents a complex task. It requires biomechanical knowledge and analytic mechanics to determine deformity that compensates in a primary plane of dominance. The purpose of the two chapters in this book is to refer to flatfoot and podological deformities and to present clinical evaluation, radiographic assessment, and mechanisms of occurrence. It also proposes surgical management for three types of flatfoot deformity as seen compensating in a dominant plane. In such cases, multiple surgical options are available to treat the underlying deformity and associated symptoms. In the discussion on the various types, biomechanical focus concerning articular geometry and its modes of compensation will be highlighted. The purpose of these two chapters is to discuss and understand the benefits of the reconstructive surgical procedures (osteotomies) for flatfoot treatment and the benefits of the arthrodesis-type procedures [11, 12].

6. Podological deformities and management

Podological deformities are the deformities that mainly occur in the foot complex. The deformities may be congenital or acquired. The commonest congenital deformities in the foot are Congenital Talipes Equino-Varus (CTEV), Vertical Talus, Hallux Valgus, Pes Cavus, Pes Planus, and Claw Toe. The acquired deformities are developed later in life, mainly due to trauma or foot fractures. In this chapter, the various conservative and surgical managements are analyzed, as also the postoperative management with the purpose of correcting the deformities, to improve biomechanical aspect and the gait pattern.

7. Functional rehabilitation after Achilles tendon rupture

Controversy continues to exist regarding optimal treatment of an acute Achilles tendon rupture, despite the research in the last decades. The proposed treatments can be classified into three types: first, conservative management with cast immobilization or functional bracing; second, operative management with open repair (with or without augmentation) and lastly minimally invasive or semi-open procedures with closed percutaneous repair (ultrasound (U/S) guidance or endoscopic control). The proposed postoperative rehabilitation protocols refer to non-weight bearing with below knee cast immobilization for 2 to 3 weeks and afterwards functional bracing for 5 to 6 weeks, and also early ankle motion exercises and partial weight bearing [13, 14].

In the chapter on Achilles tendon, the current literature concerning the management of acute tendon rupture is analyzed. It is observed that open operative treatment has a lower risk of re-rupture (1.4–5%) than nonoperative management (2.4–13.0%). In the meta-analysis of Ochen et al., it is analyzed in detail based on the systematic review that a significant reduction in re-rupture after operative treatment (2.3%) is observed compared to nonoperative treatment (3.9%) [13].

Furthermore, in the study of Khan et al., it is presented that the risk of other complications is diminished by percutaneous repair (26.1% open vs. 8.3% percutaneous group) [14]. From the meta-analysis of the literature, the clear tendency that either conservatively or operatively, early functional rehabilitation should be started as soon as possible, is presented.

Author details

Dimitrios D. Nikolopoulos
Orthopaedic Surgeon, Arthroscopist, Central Clinic of Athens, Greece

*Address all correspondence to: drdnikol@gmail.com

References

[1] Norkin CC. Joint Structure and Function – A Comprehensive Analysis. 6th ed. Philadelphia: F.A. Davis; 2019

[2] Azar F, M, Beaty JH, Canale ST. Campbell's Operative Orthopaedics. 13th ed. Canada: Elsevier; 2017

[3] Towers JD, Deible CT, Golla SK. Foot and ankle biomechanics. Seminars in Musculoskeletal Radiology. 2003;**7**(1):67-74

[4] Kulkarni GS, Jaypee Brothers. Textbook of Orthopedics and Trauma. 2nd ed. Vol. 1. New Delhi, India: Jaypee Brothers Medical Publishers; 2008

[5] Khlopas H, Khlopas A, Samuel LT, Ohliger E, Sultan AA, Chughtai M, et al. Current concepts in osteoarthritis of the ankle: Review. Surgical Technology International. 2019;**35**:280-294

[6] Drakos M, Hansen O, Kukadia S. Ankle Instability. Foot and Ankle Clinics. 2022;**27**(2):371-384

[7] Ghanem I, Massaad A, Assi A, Rizkallah M, Bizdikian AJ, Abiad RE, et al. Understanding the foot's functional anatomy in physiological and pathological conditions: The calcaneopedal unit concept. Journal of Children's Orthopaedics. 2019;**13**(2):134-146

[8] Nikolopoulos D, Sergides N, Safos G, Moustakas K, Safos P, Moutsios-Rentzos A. Large Osteochondral lesions of the talus treated with autologous bone graft and periosteum transfer. Foot & Ankle Orthopaedics. 2019;**4**(3):2473011419874039

[9] van Dijk N. Hindfoot endoscopy. Foot and Ankle Clinics. 2006;**11**(2):391-414

[10] Nikolopoulos D, Safos G, Moustakas K, et al. Endoscopic treatment of posterior ankle impingement secondary to OS Trigonum in recreational athletes. Foot & Ankle Orthopaedics. 2020;**5**(3):2473011420945330

[11] Irwin TA. Overcorrected flatfoot reconstruction. Foot and Ankle Clinics. 2017;**22**(3):597-611

[12] Henry JK, Shakked R, Ellis SJ. Adult-acquired flatfoot deformity. Foot & Ankle Orthopaedics. 2019;**4**(1): 2473011418820847

[13] Ochen Y, Beks RB, van Heijl M, et al. Operative treatment versus nonoperative treatment of Achilles tendon ruptures: Systematic review and meta-analysis. BMJ. 2019;**364**:k5120

[14] Khan RJ, Fick D, Keogh A, Crawford J, Brammar T, Parker M. Treatment of acute Achilles tendon ruptures. A meta-analysis of randomized, controlled trials. The Journal of Bone and Joint Surgery. American Volume. 2005;**87**(10):2202-2210

Section 2

Arthropathies

Chapter 2

Ankle-Foot Arthropathies

Divyashri Nazare

Abstract

This chapter will focus mainly on the commonly found arthropathies in the ankle and foot, the pathology of the disease, its diagnosis, management and goals of management. The aim of this chapter is to understand how the basic anatomy of the joint is affected in these disorders and its effect as a whole. The learning objectives are as follows: (1) Learning the basic relevant anatomy of ankle and foot, (2) Discuss the causes, diagnosis, investigations and general prognosis. (3) Understanding its impairments, and (4) Providing a framework for the treatment and rehabilitation. It will cover the commonly found congenital and acquired conditions occurring at the ankle and foot.

Keywords: ankle, foot, arthropathy, diagnosis, management

1. Introduction

About 30 bones make the structure of ankle and foot. This structure can be divided into forefoot, midfoot and hindfoot. The distal ends of tibia, fibula, talus and calcaneum make the hindfoot. The midfoot comprises of navicular and cuboid bones and the forefoot consists of three cuneiforms, five metatarsals, and 14 phalanges. The ankle joint also known as the talocrural joint is a synovial joint of hinge type. Its articular surfaces are made up of the lower end of tibia with medial malleolus, the lateral malleolus of fibula proximally and the body of talus distally. The structure of talus and the two malleoli resembles a mortise which is adjustable and provides mobility and stability. It is supported by the fibrous capsule, the deltoid or medial collateral ligament (MCL) and a lateral collateral ligament (LCL) which has three bands; anterior talofibular ligament, posterior talofibular ligament and calcaneofibular ligament. The MCL controls eversion and pronation of the ankle while the LCL controls inversion and supination. The movements at the ankle joint are dorsiflexion and plantar flexion performed primarily by the tibialis anterior and gastro-soleus respectively. Blood supply to the ankle is provided by the anterior tibial, posterior tibial and peroneal arteries and nerve supply by the deep peroneal and tibial nerves.

There are numerous joints in the foot classified as:

1. Intertarsal joint that include subtalar or talo-calcanean joint, talocalcaneonavicular joint and calcaneocuboid joint

2. Tarsometatarsal joints

3. Metatarsophalangeal (MTP) joints

4. Interphalangeal joints

The movements permitted at these joints are

1. Inversion and eversion of foot at subtalar joint

2. Flexion, extension, abduction and adduction of toes at MTP joints

3. Flexion and extension at the distal phalanges

The foot has three arches: medial and lateral longitudinal arches and a transverse arch. These arches are integrated fully with one another and enhance the dynamic function of the foot, similar to palmar arches of hand. They are uniquely adapted to serve mobility and stability weightbearing functions by dampening the effect of weightbearing forces, superimposed rotational motions, adapt to changes in supporting surface and distribution of weight through the foot [1].

2. Contents

1. Trauma

    - Ankle injuries
    - Fracture of calcaneum
    - Fracture of talus
    - Ankle sprain
    - Recurrent subluxation of ankle

2. Inflammatory conditions

    - Osteoarthritis
    - Rheumatoid arthritis
    - Tuberculous arthritis
    - Gouty arthritis
    - Neuropathic arthritis

3. Deformities

    - Congenital

        a. Club foot

b. Rocker bottom flat foot

- Acquired

a. Pes planus

b. Pes cavus

c. Hallux valgus

d. Morton's toe

e. Hammer toe

f. Calcaneal spur

4. Other

- Plantar fasciitis

- Bursitis

3. Clinical examination

History

Assessment of pain (type, intensity, nature, duration, aggravating factors, relieving factors).

Observation/inspection

- Posture
- Gait
- Attitude of limb
- Color and texture of skin
- Deformity
- Muscle wasting
- Soft tissue contours
- Bony contours and alignment
- Scars
- Swelling/oedema
- External appliances/bandaging

Palpation

- Local temperature
- Tenderness
- Muscle spasm
- Swelling

Sensory examination – superficial and deep sensations.
Movements – active and passive

- End feel
- Accessory movements

Power
Muscle girth.
Limb length – true and apparent.
Gait analysis.
Balance.
Functional evaluation.
Footwear/Assistive devices/Splints.
Radiographic examination (**Figure 1**).

4. Trauma

4.1 Ankle injuries

Lauge-Hansen classification of ankle injuries is the most widely used based on the mechanism of injury (**Table 1**).

Fractures around the ankle can also be classified as:

- Malleolar fractures or adduction-abduction fractures
- Hind foot fractures
- Midfoot fractures
- Forefoot fractures

a. Malleolar fractures: Forced abduction produces rupture of medial ligament of ankle, fracture of medial malleolus or of both malleoli. Forced adduction produces rupture of lateral ligament, fracture of lateral malleolus or both malleoli. Fracture of both the malleoli is called *Pott's fracture.*

b. Hindfoot fracture is the injury to talus or calcaneum resulting from a fall from height or forced dorsiflexion injury to ankle.

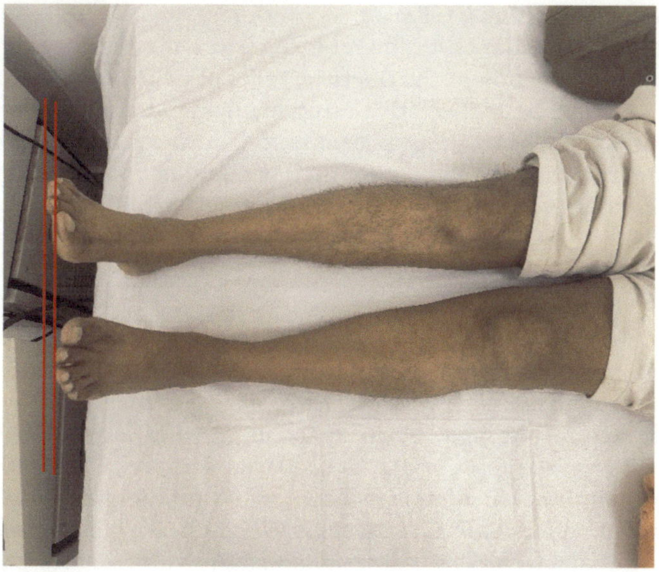

Figure 1.
Limb length discrepancy.

Type of injury	On medial side	Tibio-fibular syndesmosis	On lateral side	Others
Adduction injury	Med. Malleolus fracture with an oblique fracture line	Normal	Avulsion fracture of lat. Malleolus or Lat. Coll. Lig., Injury	—
Abduction injury	Avulsion fracture of med. Malleolus (low) or Med. Coll. Lig. Injury	Normal	Fracture of lateral malleolus at the level of ankle mortise with comminution of its lateral cortex	—
Pronation – external rotation injury	Transverse fracture of med. Malleolus at the level of ankle-mortise	Damaged	Spiral fracture of the fibula above the level of ankle-mortise or no fracture	—
Supination-external rotation injury	Transverse fracture of med. Malleolus at the level of ankle- mortise	Normal	Spiral fracture of the lat. Malleolus at the level of ankle-mortise	Fracture of the posterior malleolus
Vertical compression	Comminuted fracture of med. Malleolus, distal end of tibia and lat. Malleolus			

Table 1.
Lauge-Hansen classification.

c. Midfoot fractures: Fracture of the navicular, three cuneiform bones and cuboids usually occurs due to fall of a heavy object on the foot or in roadside accidents.

d. Forefoot fractures includes the fractures of the phalanges.

Investigations: X-ray, MRI, CT scan.

Treatment: The main aim of treatment is to restore the normal alignment of ankle mortise by accurate reduction of the fracture, relief of pain and restoration of function. The treatment can be conservative using manipulation under general anesthesia and immobilization by a below-knee plaster cast. If conservative management fails or reduction cannot resort by manipulation, then open reduction internal fixation with screws and plates is performed. After a span of 8 weeks mobilization can be initiated (**Figure 2**) [2].

4.2 Fracture of the talus

Most of the injuries are caused by fall from a height on the feet. Most minor fractures occur through the neck of talus, but in some a small chip or flake is detached. In undisplaced fractures through neck of talus, immobilization with below-knee plaster cast for 10–12 weeks is appropriate. In displaced fractures or fracture-dislocations, an open reduction internal fixation is required with cancellous screws. Then a below-knee plaster should be worn for 10–12 weeks. Weight bearing on the affected foot is avoided for the initial 6 weeks, partial weight bearing with crutches is permitted [2].

4.3 Fracture of calcaneus

The majority of fractures of the calcaneus are due to fall from a height onto the heels; thus, both heels may be injured at the same time. The weight thrust is transmitted to the calcaneum through talus thus splitting or breaking the calcaneal tuberosity. It may also shatter the calcaneus completely crushing it to pieces. A minor fracture without compression or a compression fracture is seen.

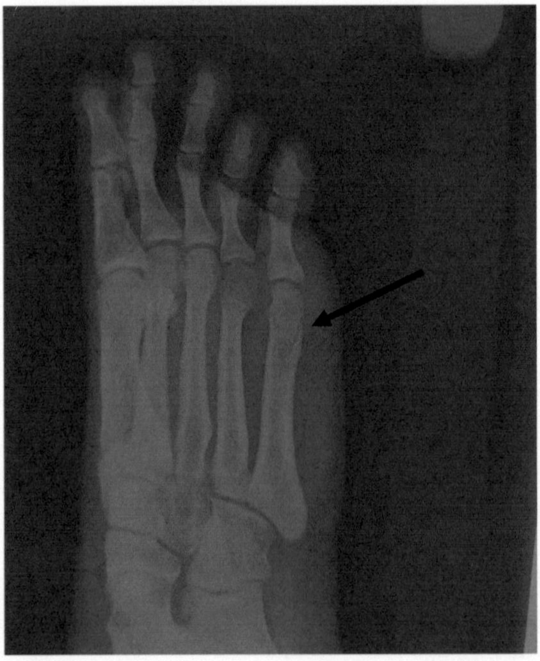

Figure 2.
Fracture of the 5th metatarsal.

Clinical features: There is severe localized pain and the patient is unable to bear weight on the heel. There is soft-tissue swelling and tenderness over the calcaneal tuberosity. Movements of the ankle, subtalar and midtarsal joints is restricted. In case of compression fracture, the heel is palpably broadened out sideways. A visible ecchymosis is seen later over the sole of the foot.

Diagnosis can be done using radiography in lateral and axial projection or a CT scan. In case of compression fracture, the upper surface of calcaneus is distinctly flattened, so that the line of the subtalar joint may form almost a straight line with the upper surface of the tuberosity.

Treatment: Protection of the heel by a below-knee plaster for 4 weeks can be done. Open reduction internal fixation in which the calcaneus is exposed from the lateral side, the fragments are levered back to their normal positions and the position is held by packing with cancellous bone grafts and application of plates and screws. Some permanent disability can occur in compression fracture [2, 3].

4.4 Ankle sprain

It indicates a ligamentous injury of the ankle. An inversion injury can cause lateral collateral ligament and an eversion force may result in a medial collateral ligament sprain. The patient gives history of a twisting ankle followed by pain, swelling and tenderness over the injured ligament. Inversion of plantar-flexed foot gives rise to severe pain and denotes talo-fibular ligament sprain. Radiological examination shows no changes in the normal anatomy.

The ankle sprain is of two types:

1. Pronation or eversion sprain: It is caused due to pronation or eversion of the foot along with internal rotation of the tibia on a fixed foot. It may be accompanied by a fracture along with a tear of deltoid ligament, tibiofibular ligament and interosseous membrane. Tenderness and swelling are present directly over the ligament. All weight bearing activities are painful.

2. Supination or inversion sprain: It is common of the two types. It occurs due to abrupt adduction-inversion force on the ankle. The tibia rotates externally on the fixed foot with the foot in supination. It causes injury to the anterolateral part of joint capsule, and one or all of talofibular, anterior tibiofibular ligament and calcaneofibular ligament.

Treatment is based on the grades of sprain:

First-degree sprain is a tear of only a few fibers of the ligament. There is minimal swelling and localized tenderness with little functional disability. It can be managed with below-knee plaster cast for 2 weeks followed by mobilization.

Second-degree sprain is where a third to almost all fibers of the ligament are disrupted. Inability to move the limb along with pain and swelling are seen. Immobilization with a below-knee cast for 4 weeks is followed by mobilization.

Third-degree sprain is the complete tear of the ligament. There is sweeling but minimal pain. It is treated using below-knee cast for 6 weeks and followed by mobilization.

Cases of partial rupture are treated conservatively with immobilization by strapping, cast brace or daily open taping. Daily taping and cast bracing helps to prevent disuse atrophy and leads to formation of adhesions. Thus, early mobilization is advised which stimulates healing of torn ligaments, improving strength and stability of the ankle joint. If surgery is performed, it is followed by a POP cast. Additionally, limb elevation to reduce oedema, vigorous toe movements, application of anti-inflammatory and analgesic drugs can be done. Cryotherapy by ice pack, ice massage or ice immersion are effective to reduce pain, oedema and inflammation. Ultrasound is beneficial in improving extensibility of the injured joints. Early mobilization by relaxed passive movements should be started as early as possible in a pain-free range. Deep friction massage is effective in reducing adhesions. Active and progressive resistive exercises should be initiated as soon as possible. Full weight bearing should be started only after 6 weeks [1–3].

4.5 Recurrent subluxation of the ankle

When the lateral ligaments of the ankle tear and fail to heal properly, the ankle may be persistently unstable with recurrent 'giving away' in which the talus moves medially in the ankle mortise. The patient complains that the ankle goes over frequently causing fall. Pain is present at the lateral side of ankle. Oedema is present with tenderness at the site of lateral ligament, the heel can be inverted passively beyond the normal range, dorsiflexion and plantarflexion remain normal.

No changes are seen in routine radiography however the talus may be fully tilted away from the tibiofibular mortise through 20° or more.

Treatment: In mild cases, strengthening of the evertor muscles is sufficient. In severe cases, operation may be required where a new lateral ligament is constructed, usually by using the peroneus longus tendon [4].

5. Inflammatory conditions

5.1 Osteoarthritis of the ankle

Degenerative destruction of cartilage is more common in the hip or knee than the ankle. It is mostly due to a predisposing factor such as a fracture, irregularity of joint surfaces from previous fracture, internal derangements, previous disease, leaving a damaged articular cartilage, mal-alignment of the joint or obesity in some cases.

It shows symptoms of pain progressing over months and years, causing limp. It may go undetectable initially. On examination, hypertrophy of the bone at the joint margins is seen. Movements at the ankle are restricted.

Diagnosis: It can be diagnosed from the history, clinical findings and radiological examination. Sclerosing at the ends of the bones is seen. Erythrocyte sedimentation rate is not elevated.

Radiographic examination: Narrowing of the cartilage space, a tendency to sclerosis of the bone adjacent to the joint, and osteophyte formation at the joint margins.

Treatment: In mild cases, often treatment is unnecessary. However, excessive stress over the joint should be avoided. Analgesic drugs, rest, supportive orthoses and in selective cases, a local injection of hydrocortisone or hyaluronate can be beneficial. Physiotherapy by shortwave diathermy and mobilizing and strengthening exercises are advisable. Surgical treatment can be arthrodesis which provides stable joint [4].

5.2 Rheumatoid arthritis of the ankle

There may be destruction of articular cartilage along with subchondral bone and pain, stiffness and deformity. The cause is unknown. It may be due to autoimmunity of the body destroying its own cells or due to an infection. Middle aged adults are more likely to be affected, women more than men. There is gradual onset with progressive worsening of pain and swelling.

Diagnosis: Rheumatoid factor is found in serum. Erythrocyte sedimentation rate and C-reactive protein are elevated.

Investigations: Rheumatoid nodules may be found in radiographic examination.

Treatment: There is no specific cure although symptomatic treatment can be given. Non-steroidal anti-inflammatory drugs (NSAIDs) and Disease Modifying Anti-Rheumatic Drugs (DMARDs) are the treatment of choice. They may provide an analgesic effect while also reducing inflammatory changes. Rest is advisable followed by physiotherapy when the symptoms reside. Occasionally, an injection of hydrocortisone can be given. Operations such as arthrodesis and replacement arthroplasty are the treatments of choice when conservative management is not helpful [4].

5.3 Tuberculous arthritis of the ankle

Tuberculous arthritis is contracted by people primarily affected by pulmonary tuberculosis. The incidence of ankle joint being affected is quite rare.

Clinical features: Children and young adults are mostly affected. The common symptoms are pain, swelling and deformity of ankle. Increased warmth, swelling and restricted movements are the characteristic features.

Investigations: The earliest change seen in tuberculous arthritis is diffuse rarefaction throughout a fairly large area of bone adjacent to the joint. As the disease progresses, the cartilage and underlying bone erodes reducing the joint space.

Diagnosis: In the active phase of tuberculosis, the erythrocyte sedimentation rate is raised. While healing, it gradually lowers. Pus culture from the abscess often reveals tubercle bacilli.

Treatment: Treatment of tuberculosis with anti-tuberculous drugs; rifampicin, isoniazid, pyrazinamide, ethambutol and streptomycin is essential to prevent further spread. In the early stages, immobilization using plaster cast or splint of the affected joint is advisable to provide pain relief and joint stability for healing for 4 to 4 months. Meanwhile, abscesses should be drained frequently. If disease progresses and the articular cartilage erodes further, a further period of immobilization and fusion of the joint is advisable [4].

5.4 Gouty arthritis

Gout is associated with disturbed purine metabolism. It is characterized by deposition of uric acid salts, especially sodium biurate or monosodium urate crystals in the connective tissue such as cartilage, walls of bursae and ligaments. Excessive consumption of purine-rich foods such as liver, kidneys, fish, seafood, beer or heavy wines are some of the underlying causes. In addition to dietary factors, comorbidities such as obesity, hypertension, metabolic syndrome, type 2 diabetes mellitus, and chronic kidney disease are contributing factors.

Clinical features: The patient is almost always over 40 and males are more commonly affected than females. Arthritis occurs in recurrent attacks, first attacking the great toe, later to the tarsus and ankle. An acute onset is sudden at night. The affected joint is severely painful, swollen, reg and glossy. Deposition of uric acid (tophi) occur at the joints.

Investigations: There are no significant changes in acute gout seen in radiography. In chronic cases, the bone ends show clear-cut erosions adjacent to articular surfaces.

There may be mild leucocytosis and elevated erythrocyte sedimentation rate. Plasma uric acid level is raised. On aspiration of the swollen joints, turbid fluid comes out.

Treatment: for acute attacks, non-steroidal anti-inflammatory drugs such as indomethacin, or naproxen can be given. Colchicine, allopurinol are sometimes used. The affected joint is rested until symptoms subside. Aspiration of effusion may be followed by instillation of hydrocortisone [4].

5.5 Neuropathic arthritis of the ankle

Neuropathic arthritis is uncommon but well recognized in the ankle, the underlying pathology being diabetic neuropathy, syringomyelia, cauda equina lesion, tabes dorsalis, leprosy, syphilis or stroke. The ankle is one of the most commonly affected joint.

Clinical features: Middle aged adults are usually affected. Swelling and joint instability are common symptoms. Pain may be present while the range of movement is restricted with significant laxity leading to instability.

Treatment: In some cases, the best treatment is to provide support to the joint with a suitable orthosis. Occasionally, arthrodesis may be performed but is difficult. The primary underlying neurological disorder should be treated [4].

6. Deformities

6.1 Club foot

Club foot is a term synonymous to Congenital Talipes Equino Varus (CTEV). It is one of the commonest congenital anomalies found characterized by plantar flexion (equinus) at the ankle joint, inversion at subtalar joint and adduction of the forefoot.

It can be classified as primary or idiopathic and secondary to paralytic disorders like polio, spina bifida, etc. It may be detected anytime since birth to late childhood.

Clinical features

1. Raised and shortened inner border of foot.

2. Exaggerated longitudinal arch.

3. Inverted and small heel.

4. Significant limitation of eversion and dorsiflexion.

5. Outer border of foot is convex and weight-bearing.

6. Bony prominences are felt on the lateral side of foot, the head of talus and lateral malleolus.

Diagnosis: Usually, in newborns the foot can be dorsiflexed so that the dorsum of foot touches the shin of tibia. This can be used as a screening test in mild cases of clubfoot.

Investigations: X-rays can be done in antero-posterior and lateral views. The talo-calcaneal angle in a normal foot is more than 35^0, but is reduced in CTEV.

Treatment: The principle of treatment of CTEV is the correction of the deformity and its maintenance. There are non-operative and operative methods to do so.

1. **Non-operative methods**: In the conventional Kite method, correction of forefoot adduction followed by heel inversion, cavus and equinus at the end is the sequence. Dorsiflexion of the foot along with pressure on the inner border of heel corrects the cavus, equinus and inversion of the heel. In children above 2 years of age, passive manipulation as mentioned above is carried out and maintained by strapping, splinting or below-knee POP cast. A Dennis Brown splint or Wheaton brace can be used.

2. **Operative methods**:

    i. Soft tissue release and external fixation: The tight structures on the medial side of foot are divided; tibialis posterior tendon, talonavicular joint capsule, tendon sheaths of long flexors, capsule of subtaloid joint, plantar calcaneonavicular ligament and origin of plantar muscles and fascia. Z-plasty is used to lengthen the Tendo-Achilles. Then the foot is immobilized in a POP cast for 4–6 weeks.

    ii. Bony correction: Triple arthrodesis or subtaloid-midtarsal arthrodesis is used for bony corrections.

    iii. Wedge tarsectomy: A wedge from the tarsus-calcaneum, cuboid and talus of the foot is removed. POP cast is applied after correction by manipulation and maintained for 6 weeks.

Physiotherapy management: Graded manipulation by passive movement is done to correct the deformity. The most important factor is maintenance of optimal alignment. Immobilization by adhesive plaster can be done in mild cases extending from the medial condyle of knee, passing under the heel to pull it into valgus and taken right up to outside of the knee. Another strip extends from the lateral malleolus, dorsum of foot, below the great toe to pull the foot into valgus position and ending on the outer side of knee. This is continued for 2 months.

Night splints or resting posterior corrective splints should be worn to prevent recurrence. Ambulatory training with maintenance of foot in corrected position should be taught [1–4].

6.2 Rocker bottom flat foot

Also known as Congenital vertical talus, this is referred to flattening of the longitudinal arch of foot. The talus is distorted plantarward and medially, calcaneus in equinus, foot dorsiflexed, convex sole with deep creases on dorsolateral aspect of foot.

Diagnosis: The deformity is seen as flattening of medial arch of foot. The sole is convex as both talus and calcaneus are in equinus and the foot is dorsiflexed at midtarsal joints. There is localized tenderness. Movements of the tarsal joints, supination and pronation, are painful and restricted. X-ray of foot is performed for investigations.

Management: It is difficult to treat this condition conservatively due to its high recurrence rate. Wedging casts, braces, modified shoes can be used for correction of deformity. Ambulatory training with optimal positioning of foot should be initiated early. Suitable footwear with or without arch support can be advised.

Surgical management can be done by release of soft tissue contractures, ORIF with Kirschner wires, Grice arthrodesis of subtalar joints, Triple arthrodesis of subtalar and midtarsal joints can be the treatment of choice. Postoperatively, the foot is immobilized in a plaster cast with foot dorsiflexed [5].

6.3 Pes planus

Also known as the Flat Foot, the deformity is characterized by depression of the medial longitudinal arch. This causes an excessive stress over the entire foot during weight bearing.

Causes: Congenital, Potts' fracture, ligament laxity, injury to the calcaneum, bony ankylosis of talocalcaneal bar, cause a flat foot even during non-weight bearing whereas peroneal spasm, rheumatoid arthritis and tuberculosis cause flattening of foot during weight bearing.

Types: There are four principal types;

- Flexible: with normal peroneals
- Rigid: with normal peroneals
- Rigid: with spastic peroneals
- Rocker bottom (vertical): position of talus distorted obliquely downward.

Clinical features: Usually except for spasmodic variety, there is no pain. However, pain may arise on weight bearing. There may be localized tenderness. The longitudinal arch is diminished. The movements of the tarsal joints are painful and restricted.

Investigations: A clinical examination and an X-ray examination in the AP and lateral views can be performed.

Treatment: In children below 3 years of age, shoes with medial arch support should be used. Custom prosthesis for children in 3–10 years of age can be used. In the later stages, a well-molded orthosis should be worn. Manipulation under anesthesia in children followed by POP cast for 2–4 weeks.

Surgical management by Triple arthrodesis is a treatment of choice as it provides a means of deformity correction and stabilization. Post-operatively, a POP cast is advised for 2–4 weeks, followed by modified shoes with arch support should be worn. Modified Hook-Miller's procedure or Durban's flat foot plasty are some other options.

Physiotherapy management:

- Strengthening and endurance exercises in warm water.
- Corrective gait training in the presence of orthoses, weight bearing on the lateral border of foot without orthoses.
- Toe curling exercises even when shoes are worn.

- Specific exercises for the medial longitudinal arch and transverse arches supporting muscles including posture correction [4].

6.4 Pes cavus

There is a significant exaggeration of the longitudinal arch of the foot with dropping of the tarsus. It is also known as contracted foot, and can be associated with equinovarus or calcaneal deformities. The paralysis of plantar flexors results in unopposed action of the dorsiflexors thus causing pes cavus. The anterior transverse arch is dropped. When the intrinsic muscles are paralyzed, their stabilizing action is lost thus causing uncontrolled action of the long toe flexors, which causes clawing of the toes. The anterior tibial muscles thus exert excessive pull, resulting in raising of the anterior part of calcaneum and depression of the anterior transverse arch with the hyperextension of the MTP and flexion of the IP joints.

Treatment: If treatment is started in the early stages with customized shoes and physiotherapy, it helps to control the deformity. In the later and neglected stages, surgical intervention is needed.

- Steindler's Operation: All the muscles below the calcaneum and the plantar fascia are divided. They slide forward and get attached to the bone distally thus correcting the cavus deformity. Then a POP cast is applied in the corrected position for 3–4 weeks.

- Lambrinudi's Operation: The arthrodesis of the IP joints corrects the clawing of toes, the long toe flexors act as support for the metatarsal heads. This helps to redistribute the muscle power in the foot.

- Fasciotomy: Plantar fascia along with the tendons of extensor digitorum longus are divided. The foot is stretched and stabilized, the deformity corrected and immobilized in a plaster cast for 3–4 weeks (**Figure 3**).

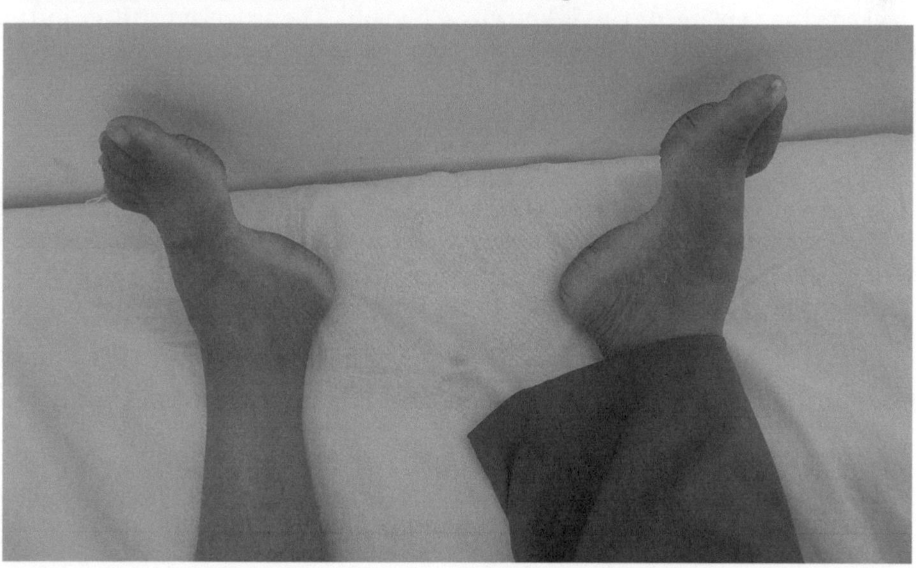

Figure 3.
Pes Cavus.

Physiotherapy management:
For conservatively managed cases

- Pain control by pain-relieving modality, faradic foot bath and exercises under warm water
- A sand bag or a weight can be placed on the dorsum of foot to maintain the contact of foot with ground. Stretching technique can be used.
- Movements such as dorsiflexion with toe extension stretches the longitudinal arch. Resisted toe extension prevents clawing of the toe.
- Corrective shoes with soft padding

For surgically managed cases

- Exercises of the joints free from immobilization
- When plaster is removed, active exercises of the ankle, foot and metatarsophalangeal joints
- Stretching of the longitudinal arch by weigh bearing and weight transfers
- Re-education of gait [4].

6.5 Hallux valgus

It is characterized by abnormal abduction of the first metatarsal with adduction of the phalanges. A false bursa may be formed over the first metatarsal head, which may be thickened and enlarged. This is known as 'bunion'. The articular cartilage inflames, erodes, atrophies. New bone forms on the medial side of the metatarsal head also known exostosis or spur. The extensor hallucis tendon is shortened and displaces laterally.

Causes: Rheumatoid arthritis, Gout, wearing pointed shoes with high heels, idiopathic, etc.

There are no other symptoms. It acts as a mechanical disadvantage thus increasing the deformity. Intrinsic muscles also cannot act effectively. These adequacies result in the dropping arch and foot eversion.

Treatment:

In severe cases, surgical management is necessary.

- Arthroplasty: The bunion and exostoses are excised, shortened and soft tissues are divided. The joint is aligned in the maximally correct position.
- Keller's operation: The excision of base of proximal phalanx with the bunion and medial portion of the head of metatarsal.
- Mayo's operation: Excision of the metatarsal head. Firm dressings or plaster cast for 2–3 weeks after surgery.

- Arthrodesis: Fusion of the metatarsophalangeal joint of the big toe.
- Mitchell's osteotomy: Osteotomy of the neck of the first metatarsal.

Mild cases can be managed by physiotherapy and proper footwear.

- Relaxed passive stretching of abduction of the toe
- Straight inner border footwear with wedge between the great toe and second toe helps in maintaining constant abduction stretch on the great toe. Night splints may be worn.
- Vigorous active exercises for the strengthening the lumbricals and interossei.
- Weight bearing on the lateral aspect of the foot to avoid pressure and pain
- Faradic foot bath to relieve pain, improve circulation and induce contractions of the intrinsic muscles.
- Active fanning of the toes in the warm water with assisted abduction of great toe.
- Gait training and ambulatory activities can be started gradually to avoid limping (**Figure 4**) [2].

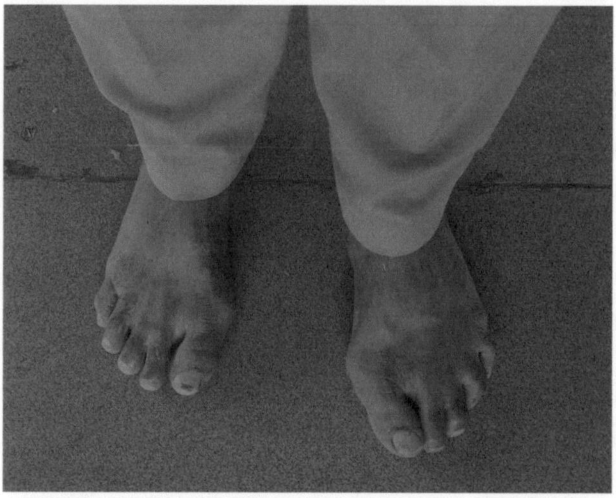

Figure 4.
Hallux Valgus.

6.6 Morton's toe

It is also termed as Metatarsalgia and defined as the deformity of foot characterized by development as neuroma, usually of the most lateral branch of the medial plantar nerve, between the 3rd and 4th, or less frequently between any two metatarsal heads.

Diagnosis:

- Pain, which increases while walking
- Disability
- Restricted and painful movements of the toe.

Investigation: X-ray of foot.
Management:
Conservative management

- Analgesics – NSAIDs, Paracetamol
- Corrective foot wear and avoid narrow toe shoes
- Gait training with metatarsalgia foot support

Surgical management: Excision of the neuroma followed by immobilization. Weight bearing after 1–2 weeks [2, 4].

6.7 Hammer toe

It is a fixed flexion deformity of the proximal interphalangeal joint and flexion or extension at the distal interphalangeal joint of the toe, usually with the hardening over the prominent proximal joint. There is usually a contracture of the second toe which may be congenital or familial in origin. Tight shoes also produce a hammer toe. The long extensor tendons contract along with the overlying skin.

Clinical features:

- Pain
- Deformity: Hyperextended MTP, hyper flexed interphalangeal and hyperextended distal phalangeal joint
- Painful and restricted movements

Investigations: X-ray of foot.

Treatment: The toe may be strapped to the neighboring toes in the corrected position with adhesive plaster or with kinesio-taping. Corrective splint (Hallux Valgus Splint) should be used even during rest to maintain constant stretch. Relaxed passive stretching helps stretch the short muscles.

Surgical management: Excision of the proximal interphalangeal joint helps to correct the deformity. In severe cases, arthrodesis of the first interphalangeal joint can also be performed. Surgery is followed by immobilization for 4–6 weeks after which weight bearing can be permitted.

Postoperatively, mobilization and stretching of the metatarsophalangeal and interphalangeal joints should be performed. Following all the procedures, maintenance of the correct alignment along with other routine procedures are adopted [4].

6.8 Calcaneal spur

Constant overstrain of the plantar fascia causes stripping of the periosteum over the calcaneum. The gap thus formed is filled up by the bony proliferation, resulting in a bony spur formation. Occasionally, a bursa may form over the bony spur which gets inflamed resulting in pain. It may be painful. It is a manifestation of the plantar fasciitis.

Clinical features: Pain, swelling, deformity, pain during walking.

Investigations: An X-ray of the foot in the AP and lateral views: Seen as a transverse ridge or bar of bone over the calcaneal tuberosity.

Treatment:

Conservative management

- Pain relieving techniques such as infrared radiation, shortwave diathermy, hydrocollator packs.
- Analgesics: NSAIDs, corticosteroids.
- Shoe with wedge or a SORCO rubber heel pad to relieve strain from the fascia.
- Faradic current to induce contractions in the intrinsic muscles, improving muscle tone, power and circulation.
- Exercises in warm water can be encouraged before initiating weight bearing.

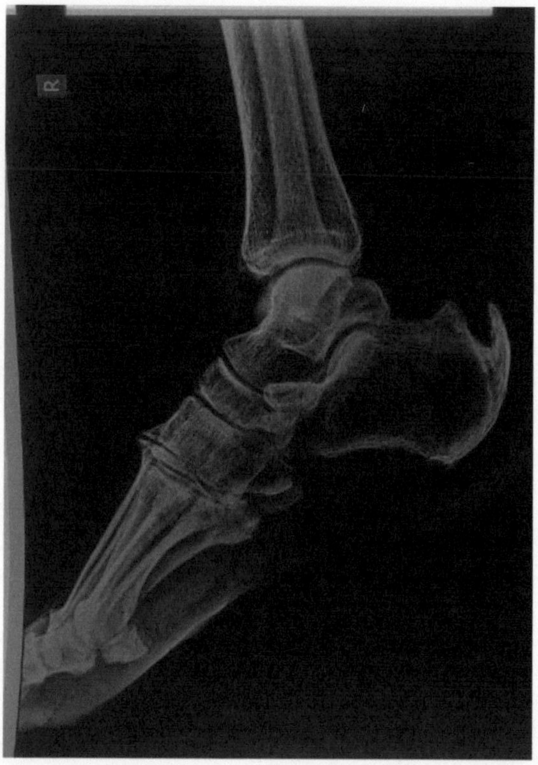

Figure 5.
Calcaneal Spur.

Surgical management: Excision of the spur can be performed if pain is persistent followed by weight bearing after 3–4 weeks (**Figure 5**) [2, 4, 5].

7. Other conditions

7.1 Plantar fasciitis

This is one of the commonest causes of heel pain.
Common causes of heel pain:

- Subtalar joint disease
- Achilles tendonitis
- Diseases of the calcaneum
- Retrocalcaneal bursitis
- Fat pad inflammation
- Calcaneal spur
- Plantar fasciitis

A repeated series of microtrauma to plantar fascia due to sustained stress of weight-bearing due to jumping, running, hopping results in plantar fasciitis. A significant amount falls over the plantar fascia stabilizing the foot from the heel raise to the toe-off phase of gait when the MTP joint are extended.

Clinical features: Pain over the inner aspect of heel or sole in weight-bearing positions. The pain is usually worse in the morning when the patient steps down from the bed or rises on the ground for the first time. Tenderness is present on palpation over the inner part of calcaneus which is the site of origin of plantar fascia.

Investigation: X-ray of the heel shows a bony spur over the calcaneum.

Treatment: A soft cushion or a silicon heel pad can be used within the shoes along with NSAIDs. A local steroid injection can be given in the plantar fascia at the tender point to relieve pain [2, 4].

7.2 Bursitis

Inflammation of the bursa is termed as bursa. It may be due to a mechanical irritation or from bacterial infection. Bursitis can be of two types:

1. *Irritative bursitis*: It is caused due to overpressure or friction and occasionally due to a gouty deposit. Inflammation of the bursa results in effusion of clear fluid into the sac or bursa. With prolonged inflammation, the sac thickens and induces pressure erosion on the adjacent bone. Some commonly seen bursitis are:

Prepatellar bursitis Housemaid's knee.
Infrapatellar bursitis Clergyman's knee.
Olecranon bursitis Student's elbow.

Ischial bursitis Weaver's bottom.
On lateral malleolus Tailor's ankle.
On great toe Bunion.

Treatment: Analgesics and rest in some cases can be sufficient along with removal of causative factor. In some cases, a local injection of hydrocortisone can be given. Rarely, excision of the bursa is required.

2. *Infective bursitis*: a bursa may become infected by a pyogenic or tubercular infection. It is commonly seen in the trochanteric bursa or prepatellar bursa. It has to be treated with surgical drainage and antibacterial drugs [4].

Bibliography

1. Adam's Outline of Fractures: Including Joint Injuries. p. 12e

2. Wooden MJ, Donatelli, RA. Orthopaedic Physical Therapy

3. Elmslie RC. Recurrent subluxation of the ankle-joint. Annals of Surgery. 1934;**100**(2):364

4. Valderrabano V, Horisberger M, Russell I, Dougall H, Hintermann B. Etiology of ankle osteoarthritis. Clinical Orthopaedics and Related Research®. 2009;**467**(7):1800-1806

5. Michelson J, Easley M, Wigley FM, Hellmann D. Foot and ankle problems in rheumatoid arthritis. Foot & Ankle International. 1994;**15**(11):608-613

6. Alpert SW, Koval KJ, Zuckerman JD. Neuropathic arthropathy: Review of current knowledge. JAAOS-Journal of the American Academy of Orthopaedic Surgeons. 1996;**4**(2):100-108

7. Rubio EI, Mehta N, Blask AR, Bulas DI. Prenatal congenital vertical talus (rocker bottom foot): A marker for multisystem anomalies. Pediatric Radiology. 2017;**47**:1793-1799

8. Yoo WG. Effect of the intrinsic foot muscle exercise combined with interphalangeal flexion exercise on metatarsalgia with Morton's toe. Journal of Physical Therapy Science. 2014;**26**(12):1997-1998

9. Schrier JC, Verheyen CC, Louwerens JW. Definitions of hammer toe and claw toe: An evaluation of the literature. Journal of the American Podiatric Medical Association. 2009;**99**(3):194-197

10. Aaron DL, Patel A, Kayiaros S, Calfee R. Four common types of bursitis: Diagnosis and management. JAAOS-Journal of the American Academy of Orthopaedic Surgeons. 2011;**19**(6):359-367

Author details

Divyashri Nazare
Mahalaxmi College of Physiotherapy and Rehabilitation Centre, India

*Address all correspondence to: hidivyashri@gmail.com

References

[1] Chaurasia's BD. Human Anatomy. 9th ed. Vol. 2. pp. 175-178

[2] Joshi J, Kotwal P. Essentials of Orthopaedics and Applied Physiotherapy. 3rd ed. New Delhi: Elsevier; 2017. pp. 212-216. 413-416, 595-599, 604-605

[3] Maheshwari J, Mhaskar VA. Essential Orthopaedics. 6th ed. Haryana: Jaypee Brothers Medical Publishers; 2019. pp. 163-166, 210-218

[4] Hamblen DL. Adams's Outline of Orthopaedics. Hamish Simpson. p. 14e. 420-421, 430-438, 440-443, 448-449, 454-462

[5] Kapoor PS. Textbook of Orthopedic Physiotherapy. 223-228, 241-248, 285-286, 323-324

Section 3

Forefoot Pathologies

Chapter 3

Perspective Chapter: Podological Deformities and Its Management

Chandrasekaran Kuppusamy, Senthil Selvam Pannir Selvam, Sandhiya Manohar, Madhumathi Kuppuraj, Sharmila Subramani, Karthikeyan Shanmugam, Jayaseelan Vijayalakshmi Kunaseelan and Manjula Subramanian

Abstract

The ankle and foot complex plays on important role in gait and weight bearing of the body weight. The deformity of the ankle and foot affects and alters the biomechanics of the body and normal gait pattern, and this consequently affects the other parts and joints of the lower limb and also trunk.

Keywords: podiatry, deformity, congenital disorder, gait abnormality, pes cavus, pes planus, vertical talus, CTEV, hammer toe, bunion deformity

1. Introduction

Podological deformities are the deformities that occur in the Ankle and foot complex. Deformity is any disfigurement or change in shape of the body part example in the foot. The deformities may be congenital or acquired. Congenital deformities that is present from the birth itself, acquired deformities are developed later in life occurs due to trauma, injuries or any pathology in the Ankle and Foot.

The commonest deformities in the Ankle and foot are Congenital Talipes Equino Varus (CTEV), Congenital vertical talus, Foot drop, Hallux valgus, Claw toe, pes planus and pes cavus. There are various surgical, conservative managements and post-operative managements are given to correct the deformities, improve biomechanical aspect and the gait pattern.

2. Ankle and foot—anatomy & biomechanics

The foot and ankle are a complex joint made up of twenty six individual bones of the foot and it has subtalar joint, talocrural joint, tarsometatarsal joint, talocalcaneonavicular joint and other inter tarsal joints. The ankle joint is one high stability role joint due to the presence of the structure called ankle mortise. The motions that take place in the ankle complex are dorsiflexion 20°/plantarflexion 55° in the sagittal plane and inversion 30°/eversion 20° in the frontal plane. When these motions occur as coupled motions to produce another movement which is known as supination and pronation. The range of motion that is available for dorsiflexion will be 10–20° and plantar flexion will be around 40–55°. The forces acting on the ankle joint bears approximately five times the body weight during stance in a normal walking phase and up to 13 times body weight during running activities.

The motions of ankle joint are produced by extrinsic muscles which has its attachment within the leg and the foot. These muscles are present within the various compartments like anterior, posterior and lateral compartment muscles. The tibialis anterior, extensor hallucis longus, extensor digitorum longus and peroneus tertius forms the anterior compartment. The peroneus longus and brevis forms the lateral compartment. The gastrocnemius, soleus, plantaris forms the posterior compartment. The deep posterior compartment comprises of tibialis posterior, flexor digitorum longus and flexor hallucis longus. The tibialis anterior and extensor hallucis longus produces dorsiflexion and inversion of the foot. The peroneus tertius produces dorsiflexion and eversion of the foot. The extensor digitorum longus assists in dorsiflexion. The peronei muscles on the lateral compartment produces plantar flexion and eversion of the foot. The calf muscles on the posterior compartment produces plantarflexion of the foot. The tibialis posterior, flexor digitorum longus and flexor hallucis longus produces plantarflexion and inversion of the foot (**Figure 1**).

The ankle joint possesses high congruency during the activity of daily living as the load bearing area is larger and has high stability role. The larger contact area in the ankle joint occurs mostly in the stance phase during normal gait. The maximum power of the ankle complex is generated around 50% in gait cycle during the forefoot rocker phase correspondingly with the force production of the plantar flexors which is required for the lower extremity to propel the body forward towards toe-off. The other form of stability for foot as a whole is provided by the presence of plantar Aponeurosis which takes up to 60% of the weight bearing and the action tie beam around 25% from the metatarsals. The toe extension during the normal gait cycle makes the plantar Aponeurosis to become taut thereby increases the ability to withstand larger amount of stress. This mechanism by several authors have been depicted as Windlass mechanism of the foot.

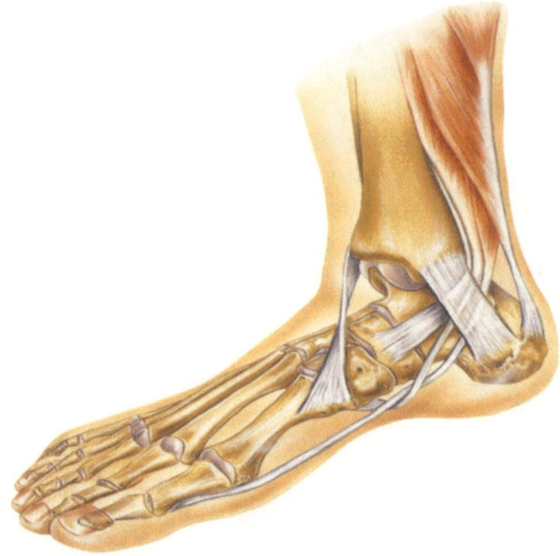

Figure 1.
Ankle and foot anatomy.

3. CTEV

3.1 Definition

The CTEV is also known as Clubfoot. It is one of the most common congenital musculoskeletal deformity occurs in children. CTEV is characterized by the fixation of the foot in adduction, supination and varus (**Figure 2**).

3.2 Etiology

The cause is idiopathic. But combination of genetics and environmental factors contribute to this condition.

Risk factors:

- Family history: Parents and siblings with same condition can have higher chance of developing disease to the new born.
- Congenital deformities: Spina bifida, cerebral palsy, or connective tissue disorders, could develop clubfoot later stages of life.
- Environment: Smoking and intake of recreational drugs during pregnancy, oligohydramnios.
- Gender: Males are like to be affected by the condition.

Epidemiology: It is more common in firstborn children and males. Incidence rate is 1:1000

3.3 Clinical features

- Heel is in equinus and small.

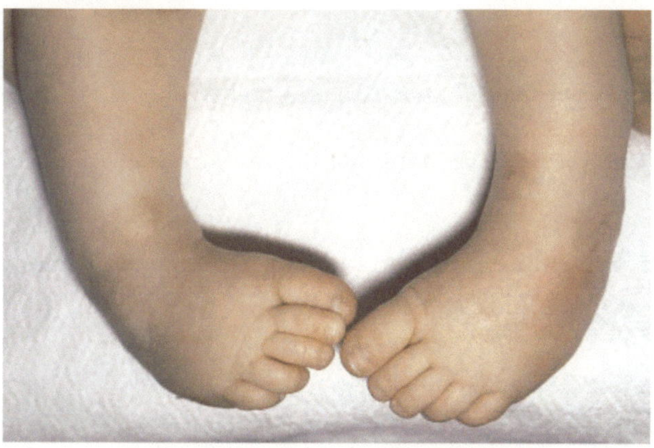

Figure 2.
CTEV.

- Foot inverted.
- Deep creases on medial and posterior aspect of foot.

3.4 Pathology

It involves four components. These component are cavus, adductus, varus and equinus where cavus and adductus deformities occurs in midfoot and varus and equinus occurs in hindfoot.

Pathomechanics: Cavus is caused due to the arch in the foot is higher than usual which causes first metatarsal being plantarflexed. The second part of the CTEV is adductus, here the navicular bone moves medially and gets dislocated from the talus. Varus is the third part of the deformity where heel is in varus in relation to tibia finally equinus causes increase in plantar flexion which leads to foot pointing downward.

Diagnosis: Antenatal diagnosis during 2nd trimester using ultrasonography.

3.5 Management

3.5.1 Conservative management

1. **At birth**: Mother of the baby is advised to manipulate the foot during every feed for 1–2 weeks before the casting begins.

2. **Infancy**: Ponseti method consists of two equally important phases: the corrective phase and the maintenance phase. *Corrective phase*: During the corrective phase the position of the foot is gradually corrected using a series of manual correction first cavus then adduction with varus followed by equinus and plaster of Paris casts, then finally a small outpatient procedure is performed to cut the Achilles tendon (tenotomy). The corrective phase usually takes 4–8 weeks. *Maintenance phase*: Following the corrective phase, the foot position should be retained in the same position. The maintenance phase involves keeping the corrected position of foot for the next 4–5 years using denis brown splint for 23 ho a day for the first 12 weeks. Then at night-time until 4–5 years old (**Figure 3**).

3. **Bracing protocol**: The brace consists of pair of CTEV SHOES: it will have straight inner border, outer shoe rise and no heel.

4. **Recurrent/Relapse CTEV**: Manipulations and casts are applied weekly followed by Re – tenotomy.

5. **Nonoperative treatment**: It includes the Stretching and adhesive strapping. French technique: sequential correction of forefoot adduction, hindfoot varus and equinus of calcaneum.

3.5.2 Surgical management

Neglected CTEV who do not respond for nonoperative method surgery is indicated surgical treatment are as follows:

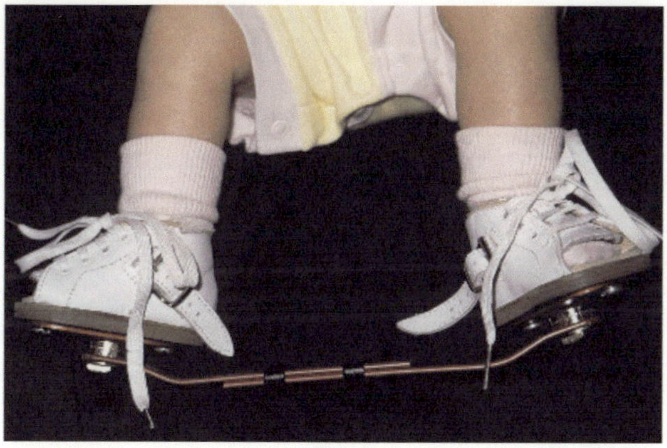

Figure 3.
Dennis brown splint.

- Turco's operation: Subtalar release along with calcaneo-fibular ligament.
- Caroll's incision: Plantarfascia release and capsulotomy of calcaneo cuboid joint.
- Cincinatti incision: It is done for posteromedial and posterolateral soft tissue release.
- Tendo achilles tendon release with posterior capsulotomy: To correct residual hind foot equinus.
- Tendon transfer.
- Triple arthrodesis.
- Talectomy.

4. Hallux valgus

Hallux valgus, commonly known as a bunion, is a deformity of the big toe joint that causes the big toe to angle in toward the second toe and protrude outward from the foot. It is caused by an abnormal balance of muscles and ligaments around the joint, which pulls it out of alignment.

4.1 Definition

The hallux valgus is a most common deformity occurs in great toe, in which the first metatarsophalangeal (MTP) joint is malpositioned, lateral deviation of great toe along with the medial deviation of first metatarsal bone (**Figure 4**).

The hallux valgus angle (HVA) is defined as the angle between the shaft axis of the first metatarsal and the proximal phalanx of the hallux (standard 15° angle).

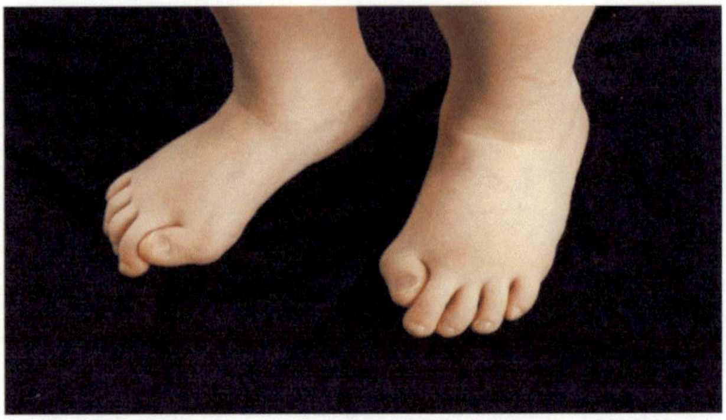

Figure 4.
Hallux valgus.

4.2 Risk factors

The various intrinsic and extrinsic risk factors causes the development of hallux valgus deformity.

- The intrinsic factors are Genetic predisposition, family history, anatomical and biomechanical factor like long first metatarsal bone, cerebral palsy, hyper mobility of the joint, severe flat foot.
- The extrinsic factors are wearing tight and pointed footwear, incorrect footwear.

4.3 Symptoms

- Pain over the medial eminence.
- Local skin or bursa irritation.
- Medial deviation of the first ray.
- Lateral deviation and pronation of the great toe.
- Pain and swelling at or near the affected joint.
- Difficulty walking or standing for long periods due to discomfort and redness or irritation around the area.

4.4 Pathology

The pathology associated with this condition includes bony enlargement at the base of the first metatarsal bone, displacement of soft tissues such as tendons and ligaments, and cartilage degeneration due to repetitive stress on these structures.

Pathomechanics: It is characterized as a combined deformity with a malpositioning of the first MTP joint caused by a lateral deviation of the great toe and a medial deviation of the first metatarsal bone. It is a deformity of the big toe joint that results from an imbalance in forces around the MTP joint. This imbalance causes the great toe to drift away from its normal position and towards the smaller toes. The main cause of this condition is over pronation of the foot, which leads to an increase in pressure on the MTP joint during walking or running activities. In addition, tight calf muscles, high heels, bunions, arthritis and genetic factors can all contribute to hallux valgus formation.

Diagnosis:

- Physical examination of the foot
- X-ray

4.5 Treatment

4.5.1 Conservative management

The HVA 20° to 45° are treated with conservatively.

- Wearing wider shoes with a lower heel.
- Using orthotic devices to support the foot.
- Taking pain medication to manage discomfort {NAIDS}.
- Physical therapy to strengthen the foot muscles.
- Steroid injection for inflamed joints.
- Physiotherapy management—These include stretching exercises, orthoses (special insoles), manual therapy techniques such as soft tissue massage or joint mobilization, and taping techniques.

4.5.2 Surgical management

The HVA more than 45° is considered severe deformity and its corrected with surgical management.

Surgical techniques includes modified McBride procedure, distal metatarsal osteotomies, metatarsal shaft osteotomies, the Akin osteotomy, proximal metatarsal osteotomies, the modified Lapidus fusion and the hallux joint fusion.

The scarf osteotomy, is a versatile diaphyseal osteotomy of the first metatarsal and is frequently used for correction of moderate to severe hallux valgus deformity.

The combination of soft tissue surgery and bony surgery followed by correct dressing and splint advised to correct the deformity.

4.5.3 Prevention

There are several ways to prevent Hallux Valgus, including:

- Wearing comfortable shoes that fit properly.

- Avoiding high heels and narrow shoes.
- Maintaining a healthy weight.
- Stretching and exercising the feet regularly.

5. Congenital vertical talus

It's the dorsal dislocation of navicular bone on the talus, the head of talus points vertically downwards and it produce rigid flatfoot deformity. Congenital vertical talus also known as Rocker bottom foot or convex pes valgus deformity.

5.1 Epidemiology

Rocker-bottom foot affects about 1 in 10,000 births and occurs equally in boys and girls. In about half of the cases the both feet are affected.

5.2 Etiology

The cause of vertical talus is unknown, however, it is often associated with a neuromuscular disease or other disorders such as:

- Arthrogryposis
- Spina bifida
- Neurofibromatosis

5.3 Pathology

The navicular bone is dislocated dorsolaterally, vertical orientation of talus bone, the calcaneum is everted and contracture of Tendo Achilles tendon. This leads to fixed hindfoot equinovalgus, rigid midfoot dorsiflexion, forefoot is abducted and dorsiflexed (**Figure 5**).

5.4 Signs and symptoms

- Rocker bottom deformity
- Equinovalgus
- Convex plantar surface of the foot
- Talar head is prominent
- Peg-leg gait

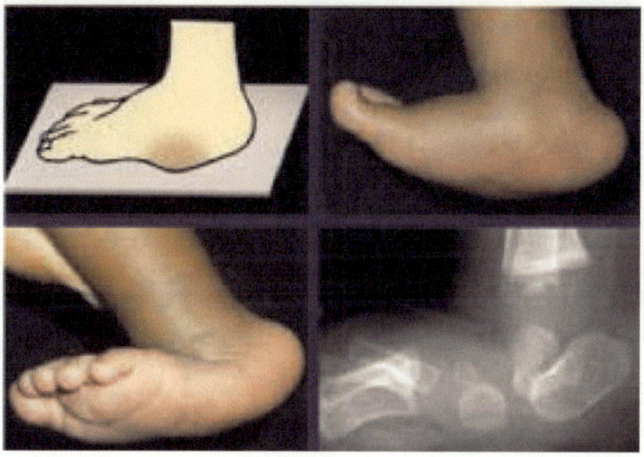

Figure 5.
Congenital vertical talus.

- Calcaneal gait
- Improper weight distribution during walking
- Balance is affected

Complications: Vertical talus can cause various complications. Following are a few of them:

- Wound necrosis
- Talar necrosis
- Under correction of the deformity
- Stiffness of the ankle
- Subtalar joint

5.5 Diagnosis

Early detection of congenital vertical talus is important for successful treatment. X-ray shows the vertically positioned talus, dorsal dislocation of navicular bone and the talocalcaneal angle is more than 40°.

5.6 Treatments

5.6.1 Nonsurgical treatment

- Manipulation
- Stretching exercises for the forefoot and hindfoot

- Casting the foot to increase flexibility
- Physical therapy exercises to stretch the foot
- Casting, bracing or stretching programs to correct the deformity

5.6.2 Surgery

Surgery is recommended at 9–12 months of age. Surgery is necessary to correct problems with the foot bones, ligaments and tendons. During the operation, pins are used to keep hones in the correct position.

The surgical procedures are:

- Soft tissue release—Lengthening of peroneal and Achilles tendon
- Reduction of talonavicular joint
- Triple arthrodesis
- Talectomy

5.6.3 Safety in surgery

Surgery can dramatically improve the long-term outcomes for your child with congenital vertical talus, but it can also be a stressful experience for you and your child. Treatment is similar to that for a congenital club-foot. Management principle are to re-establish normal relationship between bones of feet and hold them there.

6. Claw toe

A claw toe is defined or characterized as "hyperextension at the metatarsal phalangeal joints and, flexion of interphalangeal joint" [1, 2] both proximal and distal, "a foot with exaggerated arch, prominent metatarsals" [3].

6.1 Etiology

The cause of this claw foot includes either a limitation to dorsiflexion or intrinsic foot muscle paralysis or both together [3]. The exact mechanism is not known but it may occur due to the hyperextension of the MTPJ. The claw foot is seen in the following conditions. Poliomyelitis (paralysis of extensor muscle group in leg), [4], spastic spinocerebellar atrophy, hereditary spastic paraplegia, myeloneningocele, spastic spianl cord injury, multiple scelrosis (Manuel Rivera-Dominguez).

6.2 Pathology

The most common reported cause of claw toe deformity is atrophy and weakness of the intrinsic muscles caused by motor neuropathy. This causes an "imbalance between the intrinsic muscles and the extrinsic muscles that cross the MTP and interphalangeal joints. At the interphalangeal joints, the long extrinsic flexors have a greater mechanical advantage over the extensors, whereas at the MTP joint, the extensors have a greater mechanical advantage over the flexors". If the intrinsic muscles (also known as the lumbricals and interossei) are working properly, they will be able to compensate for this mechanical advantage by flexing the MTP joint while simultaneously extending the interphalangeal joints. This stabilizing action, however, is lost when the intrinsic muscles become atrophic and the extrinsic muscles become dominant. This can eventually lead to clawing of the toes (**Figure 6**).

6.2.1 Pathomechanics

"When the MTPJ becomes chronically hyperextended, the intrinsic shorten and the axis of pull shifts dorsal to the center of rotation of the MTPJ". The intrinsic are no longer able to produce a flexion moment at the MTPJ, which means that the extensors act unopposed. When the flexors are pulled to their full length, the IPJs are flexed. This clawing might be dynamic at first, and you might only notice it when you're walking. The deformity will further lead to the plantar plate tears and a subluxation develops at the MTPJ leading to the permanent deformity. The mechanism for the reverse windlass eventually breaks down, and when this happens, the toes are unable to make contact with the ground while walking, the MT heads are subjected to a greater amount of force, which ultimately leads to metatarsalgia.

6.3 Management

It is essential to have a solid understanding of, and strategy for dealing with, the underlying pathology in order to effectively lower the risk of recurrence.

6.3.1 Conservative

First and foremost, a more conservative treatment approach consisting of digital pads and footwear modification should be attempted. They are using "wide and high toe box with soft insole shoes or using an orthotic device like doughnut-shaped cushion, foamed toe cap, viscoelastic toe sleeves or toe splint".

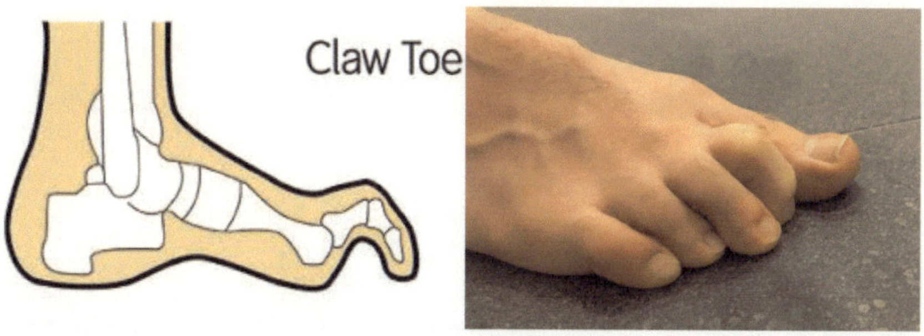

Figure 6.
Claw toe.

6.3.2 Surgical

The mild flexible form of claw toe is amenable to correction through an FDB tenotomy. A flexor-to-extensor transfer is recommended in case of hyperextension of toes at the MTPJ due to unopposed pull by the extensors and intrinsic muscle group. The Girdlestone-Taylor procedure has been used to treat claw toe deformities that can be caused by a variety of conditions. Taylor detailed the process of dividing the FDS and FDL tendons and then re-routing those tendons to the extensor aspect so that they could be sutured to the extensor expansion using a technique known as the "buttonhole" method.

7. Flat foot

Flat foot is refers to loss of the medial longitudinal arch of the foot (**Figure** 7). The flat foot is also called as pes planus. It occur either congenitally or acquired.

7.1 Pathology

The foot has the two longitudinal arches (Medial and lateral), two transverse arches (Anterior and posterior). The function of arches are shock absorption, equal distribution of body weight and propulsion of foot during gait cycle. The obliteration of medial longitudinal arch lead to flatfoot, the weight bearing area is increased, navicular bone is more prominent. Uneven weight distribution causes excessive loading on bones, soft tissues and affect walking pattern.

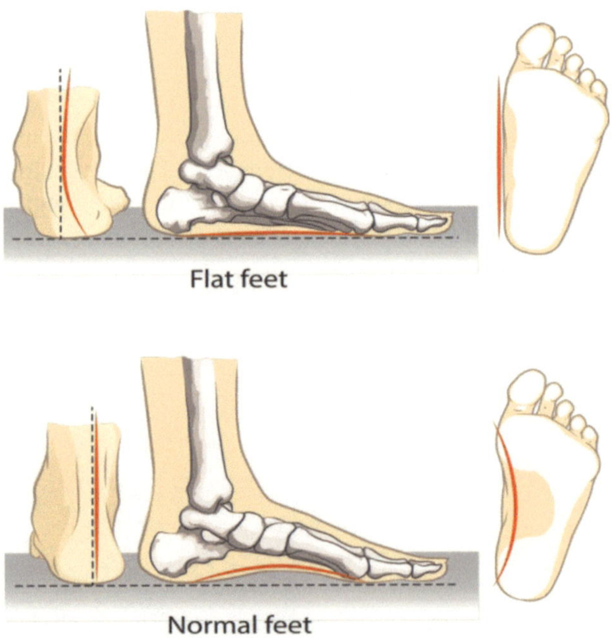

Figure 7.
Flat foot.

7.2 Types of flat foot

1. **Flexible flat foot**: During toe standing the longitudinal arches of the foot is present. During full weight bearing the arches are absent.

2. **Rigid flat foot**: During toe standing the longitudinal arches of the foot is absent.

3. **Congenital flat foot**: Present from the birth itself.

4. **Acquired flat foot:** The flat foot developed after birth.

7.3 Management

7.3.1 Conservative management

- The pain management for flat foot includes to provide the rest, activity modification, cryotherapy, massage, and ultrasound therapy used for pain relief.

- Strengthening, stretching and proprioceptive exercises.

- Footwear modification (Medial heel wedges & navicular pads).

7.3.2 Surgical management

Flat foot are corrected by reconstructive surgery. The surgeries are:

- Tendon lengthening—The Tendo Achilles tendon is lengthened.

- Tenosynovectomy—The inflamed tissues are removed.

- Tendon transfer—The affected tendon is removed and replaced by the healthy tendon from another part of foot.

- Ostetomy—It's the removing and reconstructing the bone to correct the arches.

- Arthrodesis—Fusion of the joint for better stability. Triple arthrodesis procedure commonly done to fuse all three joints in the hindfoot.

8. Pes cavus

Pes cavus is a deformity characterized by excessively high longitudinal arch of the foot (**Figure 8**).

Epidemiology: Higher in adult population.

8.1 Etiology

Factors considered influential in the development of pes cavus include:

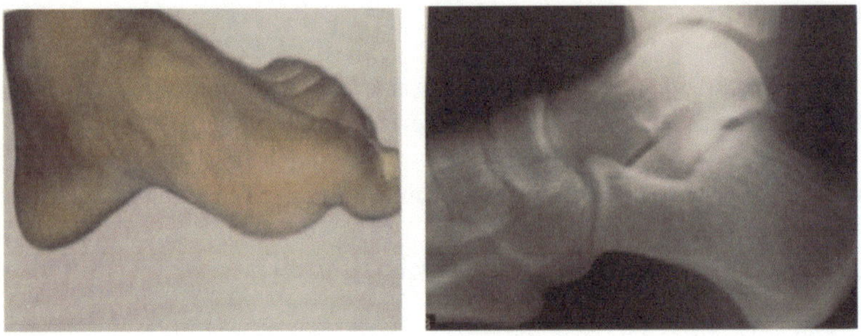

Figure 8.
Pes cavus.

- Muscle weakness and imbalance in neuromuscular disease
- Congenital clubfoot
- Posttraumatic bone malformations
- Peroneus longus tendon laceration
- Contracture of the plantar fascia
- Shortening of the Achilles tendon.

8.2 Pathology

- Weakness of intrinsic muscles of the foot.
- Muscle Imbalance—Weakness of anterior tibial muscle & calf muscle.

Pathologic anatomy:

- Dropping of the foot
- Contractures of the plantar fascia
- Varus of the heal
- Clawing of the toes.

Patho-mechanics: Pes cavus feet are often called supinated or high arched. The foot structured consists of either a high arch with a varus hind foot, a high with a valgus forefoot or both. In pes cavus, there is increased incident of ankle instability and stress fracture.

Kinematic studies of the gait demonstrated that covers feet in stance demonstrate less motion during loading response and midstance than planus or neutral foot.

This reduction in motion may result in reduced absorption of ground reaction forces and increased stress to the foot, ankle and lower limb.

8.3 Clinical features

- High medial longitudinal arch
- First metatarsal drop and pronation
- Tight plantar fascia
- Varus heel
- Clawing of toes (late feature).

Investigations/Radiography:

- Physical examination
- X-ray.

8.4 Treatment

8.4.1 Conservative management

Conservative management of patient with painful pes cavus involved strategies to reduce and re-distribute plantar pressure loading, with the use of foot orthoses and specialized cushioned footwear.

Physiotherapy management:

1. Stretching of tight muscles (peroneus longus, posterior tibialis) and strengthening of weak muscles (tibialis anterior, intrinsic foot muscles, peroneus brevis).
2. Daily manipulations, exercises, Night splints can be helpful.
3. Orthotics with depth shoes to offload bony prominences and prevent rubbing of the toes.

8.4.2 Surgical management

1. Soft tissue surgery: Tendon release in case of over pull from the muscles.
2. Jones transfer: Extensor hallucis longus is transferred to the neck of 1 metatarsal, with arthrodesis of the interphalangeal joint to improve dorsiflexion of the ankle and remove the deformity force at the MTP joint and hallux.
3. Osteotomy: Dwyer's osteotomy, Japa's V-shaped osteotomy, Anterior tarsal wedge osteotomy.
4. Bone wedge corrections of hindfoot and midfoot and triple arthrodesis.

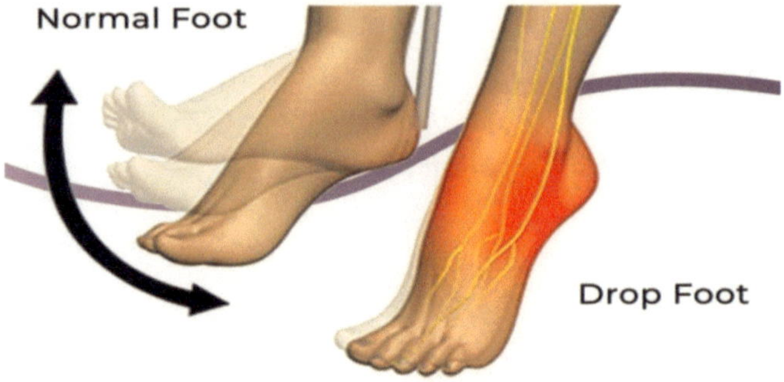

Figure 9.
Foot drop.

9. Drop foot

Drop foot is an inability to lift the forefoot due to the weakness of dorsiflexors of the foot. This, in turn, can lead to an unsafe antalgic gait, potentially resulting in falls (**Figure 9**).

9.1 Etiology

Compressive disorders: Entrapment syndromes of the fibular nerve at various locations along its anatomical pathway can lead to compressive neuropathy.

Traumatic injuries: Traumatic injuries often occur associated with orthopedic injuries as knee dislocations, fractures, blunt trauma, and musculoskeletal injuries.

Neurologic disorders: ALS (Amyotrophic lateral sclerosis).

Cerebrovascular disease (CVA).

Mononeuritis multiplex—The sciatic nerve is one of the commonly affected nerves in this condition.

Acute inflammatory demyelinating polyneuropathy (AIDP), also called Guillain-Barré syndrome.

Charcot-Marie Tooth (CMT) is a primary congenital demyelinating peripheral neuropathy and is one of the most common inherited neuropathy. It affects both motor and sensory nerves.

9.2 Pathology

The various causes lead to damage of the common peroneal nerve. The damage occur either the compression (Neuropraxia), axonotmesis, the axon is damaged, but the epineurium and perineurium remain intact. Neurotmesis is the most severe type of nerve injury. Myelin, axons, and supportive connective tissue are damaged. The injury of the common peroneal nerve leads to loss of motor supply to the dorsiflexor muscles of ankle and foot and the patient is unable to do the dorsiflexion of the foot this results foot drop.

9.3 Symptoms and sign

- Foot drop makes it difficult to lift the front part of the foot, so it might drag on the floor when you walk.

- To help the foot clear the floor, a person with foot drop may raise the thigh more than usual when walking, as though climbing stairs.

- This unusual kind of walking, called steppage gait, might cause the foot to slap down onto the floor with each step. In some cases, the skin on the top of the foot and toes feels numb.

9.4 Treatment

9.4.1 Conservative management

This includes physical therapy and or splinting and pharmacological therapy to manage pain. The goals of conservative management are to stabilize the gait, prevention of falls and contractures.

AFO (splinting): Splinting is utilized to minimize contractures. For complete nerve palsies with insufficient recovery, an ankle-foot orthosis (AFO) to prevent further plantarflexion should be ordered.

9.4.2 Surgery

The surgeries are to correct the deformity, improve the gait pattern and functional activity. The surgical treatments are:

- Nerve graft surgeries

- Triple arthrodesis

- Tendon transfer

10. Conclusion

This chapter gives us knowledge about the commonest deformities occur in the ankle and foot complex especially the congenital deformities. In this chapter discussed about the causes, incidence, pathology of the ankle and foot deformities and also the anatomical and biomechanical changes in the joint, changes in the weight distribution occur in the joints of ankle and foot due to the deformities. The various surgical procedure to correct the deformities are discussed. The conservative management like foot wear modification, positioning of the feet, orthosis and casting are discussed. Thus the chapter fully concentrated on the commonest deformities in the ankle and foot, its pathology surgical and conservative management for the deformity.

Author details

Chandrasekaran Kuppusamy*, Senthil Selvam Pannir Selvam, Sandhiya Manohar, Madhumathi Kuppuraj, Sharmila Subramani, Karthikeyan Shanmugam, Jayaseelan Vijayalakshmi Kunaseelan and Manjula Subramanian
Vels Institute of Science Technology and Advanced Studies (VISTAS), Chennai, Tamilnadu, India

*Address all correspondence to: chandrasekaran.sp@velsuniv.ac.in

References

[1] Ingram AJ. Anterior poliomyelitis. In: Crenshaw AH, editor. Campbell's Operative Orthopedics. Vol. 2. St. Louis, MO: Mosely; 1971. p. 1535

[2] Kimura T, Thorhauer ED, Kindig MW, Shofer JB, Sangeorzan BJ, Ledoux WR. Neuropathy, claw toes, intrinsic muscle volume, and plantar aopneurosis thickness in diabetic feet, BMC Musculoskeletal Disorders. 2020;**21**:485. DOI: 10.1186/s12891-020-03503

[3] Hibbs RA. An operation for claw foot. JAMA. 1919;**73**(22):1583-1584

[4] Jones R. The tretament of claw foot. Proceedings of the Royal Society of Medicine. 1912;**5**:33-36. DOI: 10.1177/003591571200501606

Chapter 4

Reconstruction of the Supple Flatfoot with the Concept of Planal Dominance

H. John Visser and Nicole Marie Smith

Abstract

Management of the adolescent and flexible flatfoot deformity represents a complex task. It requires biomechanical knowledge and analytic mechanics to determine deformity that compensates in a primary plane of dominance. This in-depth review presents clinical presentation, radiographic evaluation and mechanisms of occurrence. It also will propose surgical management for three types of flatfoot deformity as seen compensating in a dominant plane. In discussion of the various types, biomechanical focus concerning articular geometry and its modes of compensation will be highlighted.

Keywords: adult flexible flatfoot deformity, adolescent flatfoot, supple flatfoot, planal dominance, reconstructive foot and ankle surgery

1. Introduction

Although an abundance of research into the treatment of congenital flatfoot deformity has led to improved standardization of surgical options, discrepancies still exist in how surgeons best approach this common musculoskeletal condition. Differences in surgical approach appear to be based on geographic location and training. Controversy of opinion still remain on whether planal dominance actually exists (**Figure 1**). The chief author's approach tends to the theory of Root and Weed [2]. This chapter will offer insight into flatfoot deformity that is predominant in either the frontal, transverse or sagittal planes. While deformity certainly overlaps into the three planes, dominance in a primary plane often exists. The foot follows the analytic mechanical effect of Cardan coupling. A universal joint connecting rigid shafts whose axes are inclined to each other. The presentation provided will embed a stepwise approach to assess a patient clinically, radiographically and biomechanically. This will determine the surgical procedures necessary to best benefit their anatomy. This will occur once conservative measures have failed.

2. Arches of the foot

There are three main arches of the foot (**Figure 2**). The first represents the medial longitudinal arch. It is constructed of three joints: talonavicular (TN),

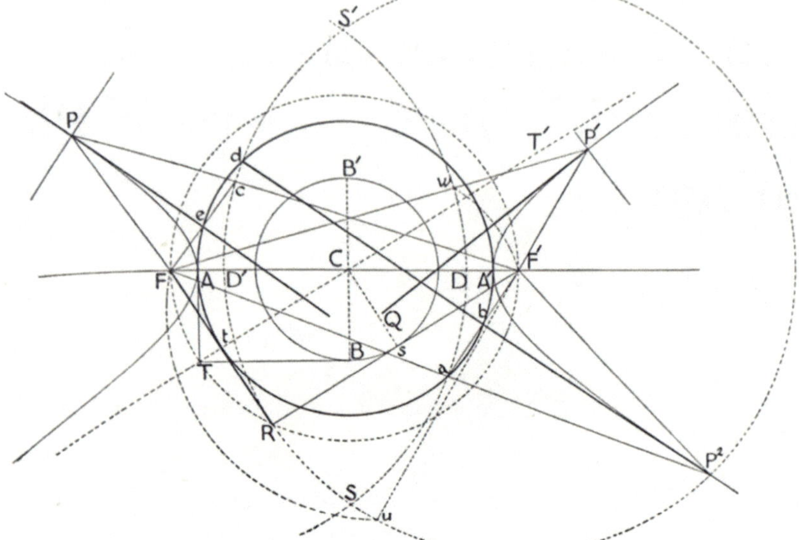

Figure 1.
Represents the complex geometry of planal dominance [1].

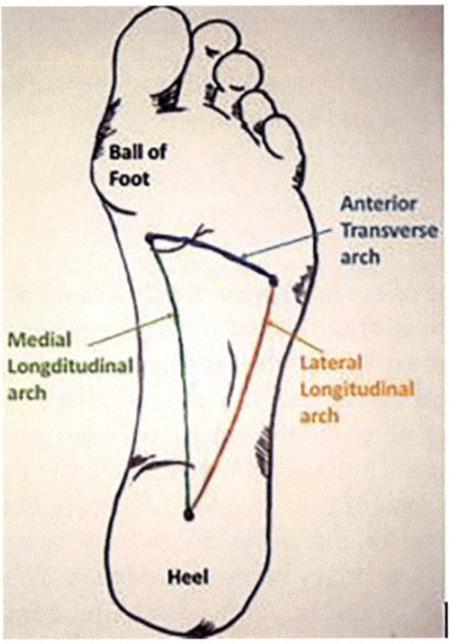

Figure 2.
Graphic depiction of the three arches of the foot.

navicular-medial cuneiform joint (NC) and first metatarsal-medial cuneiform joint (first met-MC). The second is represented by the lateral longitudinal arch. It is composed of the tarsometatarsal (TMT) four and five joints as well as the calcaneo-cuboid joint (CC). Third, the anterior transverse arch, or Roman arch, created by the metatarsals one through three and their respective cuneiforms and metatarsals four, five and their articulations with the cuboid.

DOI: http://dx.doi.org/10.5772/intechopen.110881

The medial longitudinal arch consists of two tri-planar axial joints. The TN joint which biomechanically composes the longitudinal midtarsal joint (LMTJ) axis. It deviates 15 degrees from the transverse plane and nine degrees from the sagittal plane. Thus, it provides primarily frontal plane motion. It also consists of the first-met MC joint, articulating with the navicular. This represents the first ray. It angles 45 degrees with both the frontal and sagittal planes and only slightly from the transverse plane. It thus allows primarily biplanar motion. These become effected at forefoot load (at 15% of the gait cycle) and influenced by the ankle and subtalar joints.

The lateral longitudinal arch is composed of TMT 4,5 joints as well as the CC joint. The fourth metatarsal cuboid moves only in the sagittal plane. The fifth metatarsal cuboid TMT 5 represents only motion of the fifth metatarsal. It angles 20 degrees from the transverse plane and 35 from sagittal plane. Thus, it exhibits primarily two planes of motion in equal amounts in the frontal and sagittal planes despite being a tri-planar axis. Of note the central three metatarsal cuneiform joints move according to subtalar joint and midtarsal joint motion. Whereas, the fifth ray is completely independent of their (subtalar joint and midtarsal joint motion).

The CC joint composes the oblique midtarsal joint (OMTJ) axis. It deviates 52 degrees to the transverse and 57 degrees to sagittal plane. Thus, it allows primarily motion in those two planes despite being tri-planar joint.

The anterior transverse arch (or Roman arch as it has been described) represents the TMT 1,2,3. These move minimally in the sagittal plane. They serve to provide inherent stability to the anterior arch of the foot. The lateral portion of the Roman arch remains mobile via fifth ray motion and adapts the lateral midfoot to terrain.

3. Classification of adolescent and adult flexible flatfoot deformity

This discussion will attempt and limit to classify flatfoot deformity in an adult or adolescent that exists only in a flexible deformity. There are no associated signs of neuromuscular (NM) weakness present. Intrinsic joint instability due to axis alteration is a dominant factor. Borrelli and Smith [3] discussed the flexible flatfoot from a planal dominance point of view. The authors described three planes of dominant deformity. Their discussion noted primary frontal plane compensation as STJ subluxation. The STJ is the articulation of the talus and calcaneus. It is also known as a peritalar joint articulating with the navicular as well. Thus, it composes the two tri-planar axes of the STJ and LMTJ as a peritalar complex. Axis deviation altering articular geometry creates intrinsic joint instability. Heel valgus is the primary deformity and arch flattening leads to weight bearing over the NC joint.

Transverse plane dominance was discussed as a lateral column deformity characterized by increased forefoot abduction. As will be seen, the deformity can either be affected at the STJ or OMTJ itself. In either case arch height loss occurs over the NC joint.

The medial portion TMT 1,2,3 of the transverse arch is a stable and relatively rigid articular structure. Disease and injury can lead to abnormal joint instability. The first met MC becomes unstable and thus exhibits abnormal clinical motion creating a midfoot flatfoot with loss of arch height. Weight bearing thus is primarily centered at the medial cuneiform (1st met-MC). STJ and MTJ compensation is normally not effected.

Sagittal plane deformity was defined by medial column subluxation. In this case the talus within the peritalar complex is oblique and subluxed with the talar head being weight bearing at the collapsed medial longitudinal arch.

4. Frontal plane flatfoot deformity

4.1 Biomechanics of the frontal plane flatfoot deformity

In the case of normal biomechanical function of the STJ, the axis deviates 42 degrees to the transverse plane and 16 degrees to the sagittal plane as well as 46 degrees to the frontal plane. It is known that the joint axis is determined by joint geometric anatomy. This indicates frontal plane motion signified clinically by calcaneal eversion, and transverse plane motion noted by talar adduction related nearly 1:1. Sagittal plane motion is much less and presented as talar plantarflexion.

Chambers in 1946 [4] discussed the concept of unsaddling of the STJ. He noted that the posterior, anterior and middle facets were synchronized in their movement and acted like gears. The articular surface geometry is determined by the axis. The talus moves as a cog relative to the calcaneus. In a normal state of function talar movement is determinant by an osseus restraining mechanism. Sigrid Zitzlsperger, MD described this mechanics as self-locking wedges [5]. The talar concave and calcaneal convex surfaces at the posterior, anterior, and middle facets determine talar movement. Beginning as congruous during biomechanical function talar adduction, plantarflexion and calcaneal eversion ultimately become incongruous and thus (lock) preventing further talar motion. This relates to the first 25% of the gait cycle where maximal pronation occurs and the calcaneus everts to six degrees.

When in a pathologic state and the axis becomes deviated more to the frontal plane (less vertical) calcaneal eversion (greater than 20 degrees) will exceed talar adduction. The joint structures (posterior, ant, middle facet) will fail to lock and thus a loss of the osseus restraining mechanism and failure of the self-locking wedges occurs. The end result is the supporting structures (cervical, interosseus and spring ligaments) attempt to restrain talar movement and become strained. Talar movement does not stop until the talar lateral process abuts into the floor of the sinus tarsi. Thus, as the foot proceeds to 50% of the gait cycle it fails to resupinate.

Bruce Sangeorzan, MD and colleagues only recently discussed the "forward movement of the talus" moving like a screw [6]. This factor of the talus sliding forward on the calcaneal facets correlates to radiographic findings that will be discussed. The severity of this movement is determinant upon pathologic compensatory factors such as equinus and torsional forces.

Clinically heel valgus then exceeds the normal six degrees. The forefoot loads at about 10% of the gait cycle. Normally the TN joint and LMTJ axis compensates for the heel valgus by six degrees of inversion. In cases of excessive heel valgus (greater than six degrees), further forefoot compensation will occur at the first met MC/navicular first ray. This is signified as an NC break and elevation of the first metatarsal in reference to the second (Seiberg index). Also further compensatory forces (equinus) strain the soft tissue about the TN joint allowing further motion. This is the concept of forefoot supinatus. This will be discussed in more detail in radiographic analysis. In essence, the foot fails to resupinate and thus at propulsion fails at toe off.

4.2 Radiographic evaluation of the frontal plane flatfoot deformity

When viewing the dorsal plantar (DP) view (**Figure 3A**), the talo-calcaneal (TC) angle, or Harris-Beath angle is increased. Uncoverage of the talar head varies from 30 to 50% while cuboid abduction angle remains normal. This can be explained by the talus adducting and moving forward and does not use the navicular for lateral rotation.

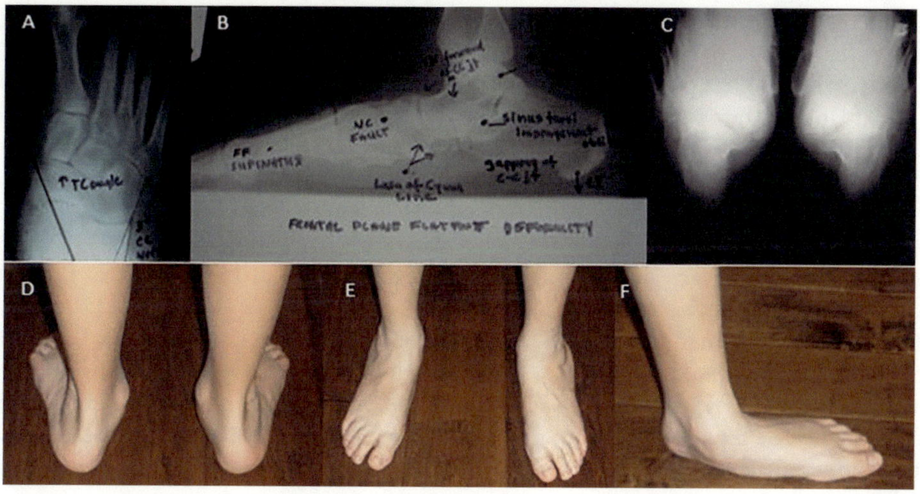

Figure 3.
A: DP view of a right frontal plane flatfoot; B: Lateral view of a right frontal plane flatfoot with annotated anatomical anomalies; C: Axial view of a frontal plane flatfoot; D: Clinical photograph showing the posterior view of frontal plane flatfeet; E: Clinical photograph showing the front view of frontal plane flatfeet; F: Clinical photograph showing the lateral view of left frontal plane flatfoot.

On the lateral view (**Figure 3B**), various radiographic deviations are noted. First one notices the orientation of the posterior facet. It is angled about 75 degrees to the weight bearing surface with the STJ axis being less vertical and more perpendicular to the frontal plane. It can be viewed as a "pogo-stick" pulling the posterior facet into that position tilting the entire talus forward, medial and down. We also see obliteration of the sinus tarsi. This is due to a lateral process abutment that led to stoppage of talar movement.

The talar declination angle is increased due to the adducted plantarflexed and forward movement of the talus. Calcaneal inclination is also decreased. This is due to the forward position of the talus over the sustentaculum tali (STT) with weight bearing forces pushing it downward. With associated gastrocnemius soleus equinus contracture it pulls the posterior tuber superior and the anterior portion of the calcaneus inferiorly. An anterior break of the Cyma line is seen. Inferior plantar gapping of the CC joint represents excessive calcaneal eversion as the calcaneus moves away from the cuboid.

At the midfoot level the presence of an NC fault is noted. As has been described this represents pathologic compensation for excessive heel valgus. This is an osseous adaption and attributes to forefoot varus. At the forefoot level, forefoot supinatus is noted. This represents piling of the metatarsals so when viewed they all appear to be on the same plane. With excessive equinus forces the TN joint is subluxed on the frontal plane due to increased inversion forces that affect the capsuloligamentous structures. The navicular, three cuneiforms and three metatarsals become aligned with metatarsal 4 and 5. This represents a soft tissue contracture.

On the axial view (**Figure 3C**) we note the talus subluxed medially on the STT. There is sloping and hypoplasia noted. This is due to the anterior talar subluxatory weight bearing forces. This then produces functional adaptation along the lines of force as described by the Law of Wolff [7]. There is then an obvious loss of parallelity between the anterior, medial, and posterior facets. Also, the calcaneal body is in valgus in relation to the weight bearing line of the tibia.

4.3 Clinical evaluation of the frontal plane flatfoot deformity

When viewing the patient from behind (**Figure 3D**) we see excessive amounts of heel (calcaneus valgus). Also noted is medial bulging of the talus and of note it is not weight bearing. A positive Helbing's sign is also seen with lateral orientation of the Achilles tendon insertion.

On the frontal view of the patient (**Figure 3E**), one notes a "reverse peek-a-boo heel sign." With the lateral aspect of the calcaneus clearly visible due to excessive heel valgus. Also note the lack of forefoot abduction due to forward migration of the talus and lack of rotatory contact with the navicular.

When viewing the foot from the lateral view (**Figure 3F**), significant collapse of the medial longitudinal arch is noted. One can clearly see the weight bearing center of rotation axis (CORA) of collapse centers at the medial-cuneiform -navicular joint (MCNJ) with the navicular tuberosity being the apex of weight bearing. Talar bulge is noted and significant but does not represent the weight bearing CORA of the longitudinal arch collapse.

4.4 Surgical management of the frontal plane flatfoot deformity

4.4.1 Gastrocnemius and Achilles tendon contracture

The approach begins first by assessing the deforming forces of the Achilles tendon contracture. The Silverskold test is utilized. If contracture exists with the knee extended and eliminated when the knee is flexed, contracture of the gastrocnemius is present. This is best approached by gastrocnemius recession. A Strayer or Baumann type of aponeurotic release is performed. If, however the contracture persists when

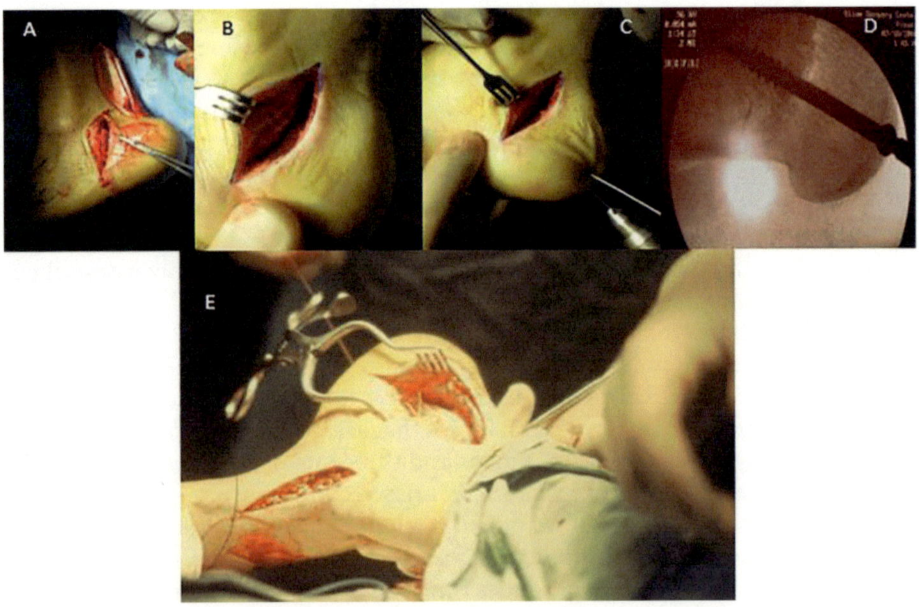

Figure 4.
A: Depicts and open z-plasty proximally; B–D: Koutsogiannis osteotomy to stabilize STJ in a frontal plane flatfoot patient; E: Gleich-Dwyer calcaneal osteotomy.

the knee is flexed it is representative of an Achilles tendon contracture. This is best addressed either open, frontal or z-plasty lengthening (**Figure 4A**), or more commonly percutaneous length by a Hoke technique. Two medial and a central lateral incision is utilized cutting 1/3 of the tendon at each site. In cases of primary gastrocnemius contracture a two incision percutaneous approach to the Achilles tendon can be utilized bringing the ankle only to 90 degrees. One must also be aware of the presence of an osseus equinus. This can be best evaluated on a lateral view looking for tibiotalar impingement lesions or flattening of the dome of the talus.

4.4.2 Posterior calcaneal osteotomy

Once the deforming force from the Achilles tendon is addressed, one then turns to the STJ malalignment. The first option is the cresentic calcaneal osteotomy described by Koutsogiannis [8]. Despite being a translated medial in the transverse plane, it allows significant correction in the frontal plane addressing the heel valgus deformity (**Figure 4B**). It has four primary biomechanical effects: 1. it converts the Achilles tendon insertion from a pronator to a supinator; 2. it aligns the calcaneal tuberosity to the STT; 3. by medial reposition it institutes gravitational forces that create closed kinetic chain supination and thus external leg rotation; and 4. its main biomechanical effect is that it displaces STJ motion by reducing pronation. On a maximal pronation force to the STJ the heel remains vertical. Thus it "displaces" the range of motion but has no effect on altering the STJ axis. The Gleich-Dwyer calcaneal osteotomy is done through the calcaneal body via a medial approach and allows a significant corrective force in the frontal plane. It can be done laterally where a medial wedge is cut in the medial side of the calcaneus (**Figure 4C**).

4.4.3 STJ arthroeresis

The second option to address STJ malalignment in the frontal plane, is utilization of STJ arthroeresis. Voegler [9] originally described arthroeresis into three separate categories (**Figure 5A–C**).

The first is "self/locking wedges" (**Figure 5A**) which represent the most common of arthroeresis implants. They are cylindrical implants that are inserted into the canalis tarsi. They serve to center the calcaneus in a vertical position in reference to the ankle joint. They also resaddle the talus into the STJ mortise. Thus while preserving supinatory motion they restrict pronation significantly. This is noted clinically by decreased calcaneal eversion, talar adduction as well as PF and forward migration of the talus. This form of arthroeresis provides corrective force to the STJ and alters its axis. In the past this was addressed with opening-wedge type osteotomy directed at the STT (anterior and middle facet).

The Selakovich opening wedge osteotomy (**Figure 5D**) was performed at the sustentaculum level. It served to reposition the anterior and middle facets parallel to the weight bearing surface and re-establish talar head support. The Baker and Hill opening wedge osteotomy of the posterior facet (**Figure 5E**) was created when it was noticed with STJ correction when performing an extra-articular Grice arthrodesis on a young patient with cerebral palsy a large gap was noted at the level of the posterior facet. Thus, rather than performing the arthrodesis they embarked with an opening wedge osteotomy of the posterior facet and restored its congruency. Both of these osteotomies serve to alter the axis of the STJ and re-established its locking mechanism.

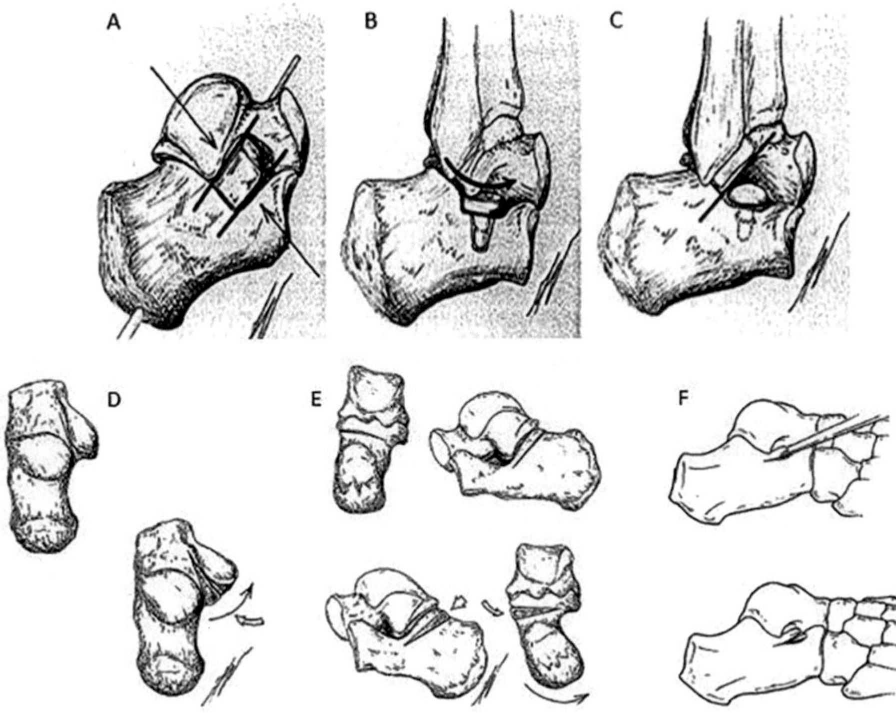

Figure 5.
A–C: depict the Vogler classification for three arthroeresis options; D: diagram of Selakovich opening wedge osteotomy of the sustentaculum tali; E: diagram of posterior facet osteotomy with bone graft as described by Baker and Hill; F: diagram of chambers procedure demonstrating application of arthroeresis concept with use of bone graft.

The second implant type is the axis altering represented by the Smith Subtalar Arthroeresis (STA) peg (**Figure 5B**) [10]. Based on the Chambers procedure (**Figure 5E**) it is placed in front of the posterior facet where it is notched at 90 degrees to the anterior portion and thus raised the floor of the sinus tarsi. It then serves to restrict talar pronatory motion and restores the posterior facet locking mechanism.

The third type of arthroesis implant are the blocking devices (**Figure 5C**). Smith altered his STA peg to have an inclined anterior thickness to block the talus in adduction by "jamming" the lateral process. Pisani [11] placed a 3.5 mm screw in front of the lateral process in the floor of the sinus tarsi. The STJ was placed in its corrected neutral position and screw placed perpendicular in front of the lateral process. In essence, all three types of arthroesis implants lead to axis alteration in the adolescent. Functional adaption of the anterior, middle, and posterior facets then occurs along the lines of corrective forces as described by Wolff.

Once the STJ is stabilized in the frontal plane, one then turns to address the medial longitudinal arch (medial column changes). As stated prior an NC fault is seen as a persistent fault in the frontal plane. This is a result of compensation for equinus and heel valgus. In cases where the fault appears subtle, a "reverse Coleman block test" may be utilized (**Figure 6A**). With this test, blocks are placed under the forefoot and the amount of block height needed is to bring the calcaneus to a vertical position. A lateral X-ray is taken and a fault if present will be clearly demonstrated.

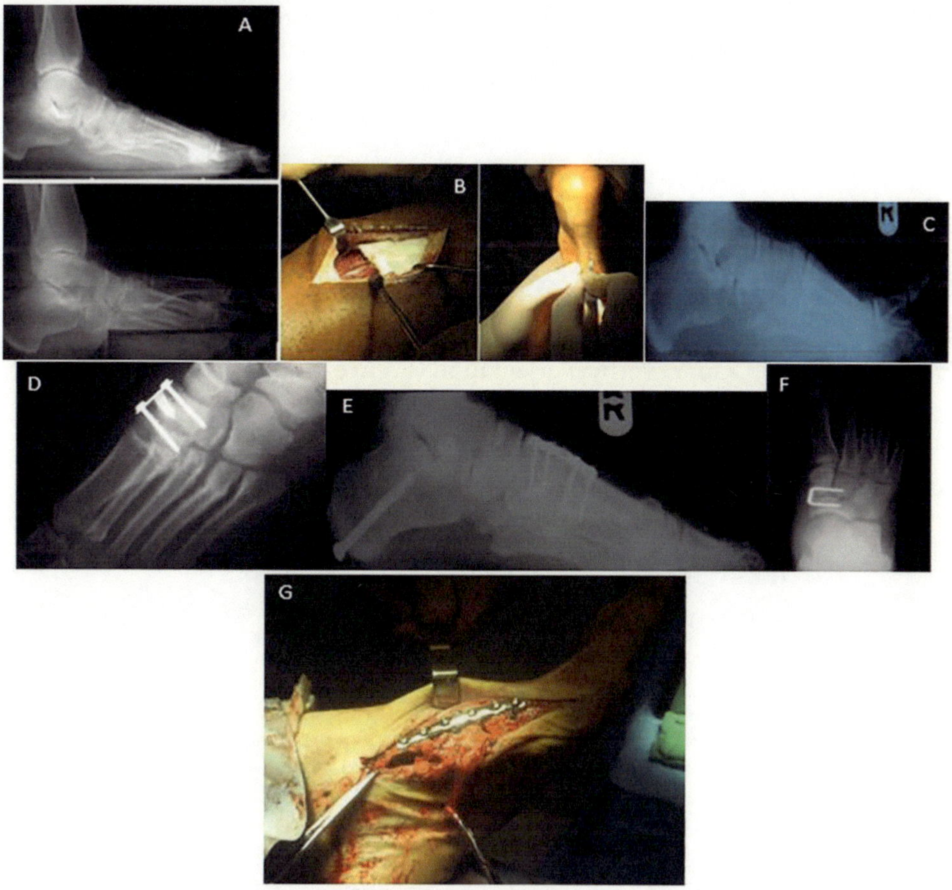

Figure 6.
A: reverse Coleman block test used to assess the presence of medial column fault. Block placed under the forefoot to identify NC fault; B: surgical approaches addressing equinus present in a frontal plane flatfoot patient; C: Jack test on a right foot to activate the windlass effect; D–F: cotton osteotomy, Lapidus, hoke navicular trans cuneiform fusion; G: Miller procedure.

In the adolescent and some adults the NC fault can be corrected by Achilles/gastrocnemius lengthening and STJ stabilization (**Figure 6B**). These procedures address the forefoot supinatus component. In these cases, functional adaption at the NC joint has not occurred. Another way to determine this condition pre-operatively is to perform Jack test (hallux dorsiflexion creating a windlass mechanism action) (**Figure 6C**).

If the NC fault present on the pre-operative weight bearing x-ray reduces, then there is no need to perform a medial column procedure. In cases where the NC fault persists on performance of the Jack test (first ray compensation), functional adaption occurs by sagittal compression forces about the dorsal portion of the NC joint. Thus, a true forefoot varus is present.

In these cases a cotton osteotomy (opening wedge of MC) or a plantarflexory MC (Mosca) osteotomy is performed. Also, the Hoke type navicular cuneiform fusion which includes the intercuneiform joint is an option. This can also be incorporated with wedging to address additional forms of forefoot abduction. The sagittal plane Lapidus procedure can be considered in the adolescent and addresses the NC fault.

It can also be also utilized as a tri-planar correction in the presence of associated hallux abducto valgus deformity (**Figure 6D–F**). A Miller procedure (**Figure 6G**) is considered in the case of a longstanding severe equinus and heel valgus. This can lead to a combined medial fault involving the NC and first met-MC joints.

5. Transverse plane flatfoot deformity-subtalar type

5.1 Biomechanics of the transverse plane flatfoot deformity-subtalar type

In the case of the transverse plane dominated flatfoot deformity we see the axis (facet geometry) in a more vertical orientation (**Figure 7**). In this case transverse

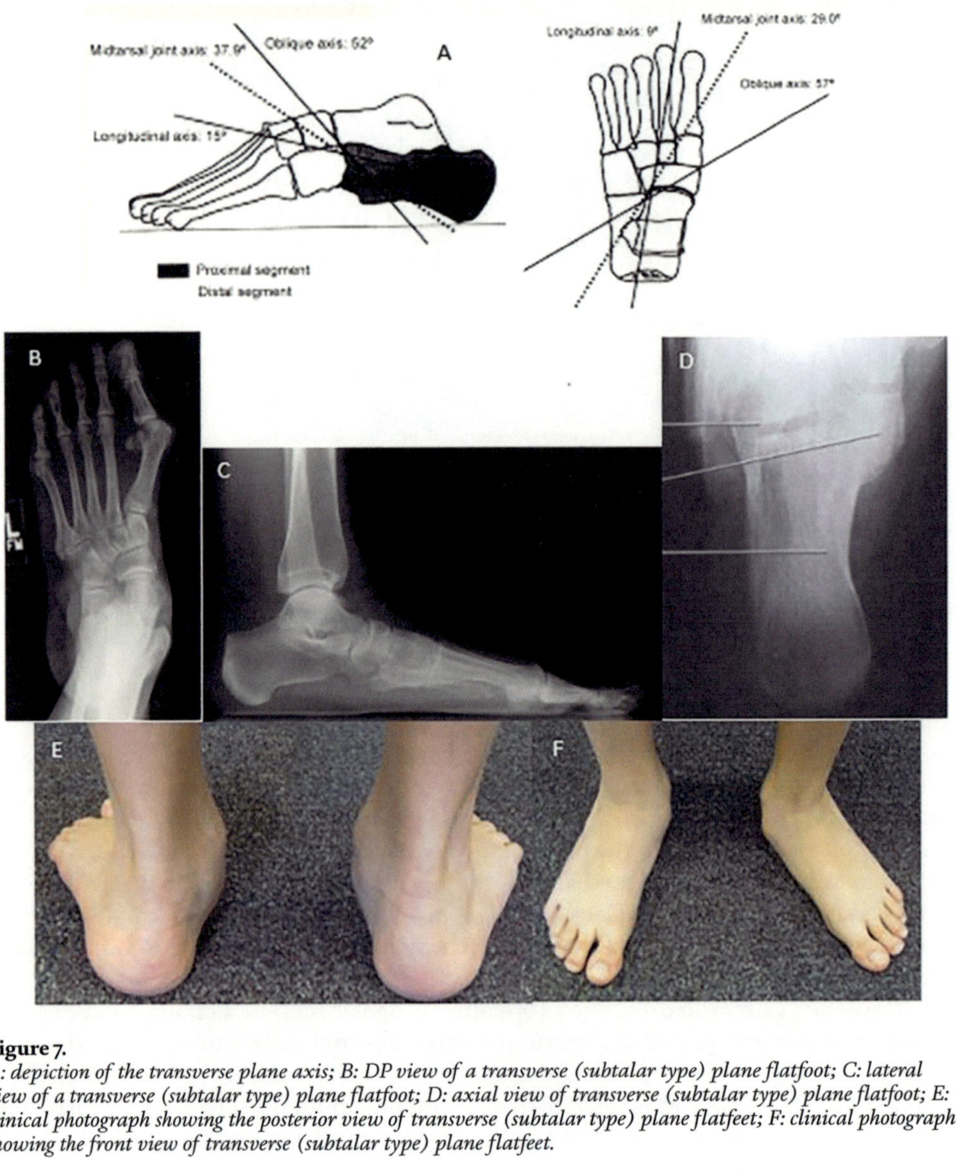

Figure 7.
A: depiction of the transverse plane axis; B: DP view of a transverse (subtalar type) plane flatfoot; C: lateral view of a transverse (subtalar type) plane flatfoot; D: axial view of transverse (subtalar type) plane flatfoot; E: clinical photograph showing the posterior view of transverse (subtalar type) plane flatfeet; F: clinical photograph showing the front view of transverse (subtalar type) plane flatfeet.

plane (talar adduction) exceeds frontal plane calcaneal eversion. The predominant deformity is forefoot abduction. There are two separate etiologies that lead to excessive forefoot abduction.

The first is generated the subtalar joint level. In this case, a significant amount of talar adduction occurs noted with an increase in the TC angle. However, the lateral column of the MTJ CC joint remains normal indicating that forefoot abduction is occurring about lateral translation of the navicular. Heel valgus occurs but remains in the 10–12 degree range. When viewing the lateral view an NC break is noted but is mild and reactant to equinus and heel valgus.

5.1.1 Radiographic evaluation of the transverse plane flatfoot-subtalar joint type

When evaluating the DP view there is a noted significant increase in the TC angle (Harris Beath) (**Figure 7B**). However, there is no sign of an increase in cuboid abduction (CA) angle. On the lateral view (**Figure 7C**) there is a paradox as there is a mild NC break but Meary's angle appears as normal. To explain this one can see the posterior facet (a more vertical axis) appears more parallel to the weight bearing surface. When using the pogo-stick is appears more perpendicular to the weight bearing surface. As the talus thus goes through its excess adduction motion the anterior and middle facets being more parallel to the posterior facet is supported through its full range of motion on the axial view image (**Figure 7D**). There is minimal PF and forward movement noted.

5.1.2 Clinical presentation of the transverse plane flatfoot-subtalar joint type

When viewing the patient from behind (**Figure 7E**) one can see a lesser amount of heel valgus at about 10 degrees. Talar bulge is noted. Also, the classic "too-many-toes sign" is present signifying increased forefoot abduction. When viewing the patient from the front (**Figure 7F**), one can see a significant amount of talar bulge but it is not weight bearing. As can be seen with a more vertical STJ large increases in talar adduction are accommodated by the STT in rotation of the navicular as well as the remaining forefoot occurs. The arch is lower but weight bearing CORA occurs at the NC joint.

5.2 Biomechanics of the transverse plane flatfoot deformity-midtarsal type

In the second case, forefoot abduction is generated at the midtarsal joint level or CC (OMTJ). In this case as the talus moves into its locked adducted position the OMTJ becomes unlocked. The result is that forefoot abduction occurs primarily about that joint. The talus "locked" into the ankle mortise leads to prominence of the medial malleolus. This is created by closed kinetic chain pronation. There is a small amount of heel valgus (approximately eight to ten degrees) and associated equinus contracture, that serves to flatten the longitudinal arch about the NC joint. Also, the dorsiflexion component about the CC joint serves to lower the lateral portion of the longitudinal arch.

5.2.1 Radiographic evaluation of the transverse plane flatfoot-midtarsal type

When viewing the DP view (**Figure 8A**), again an increase in the TC angle is noted but there is also a significant increase in the CA angle. A paradox exists with

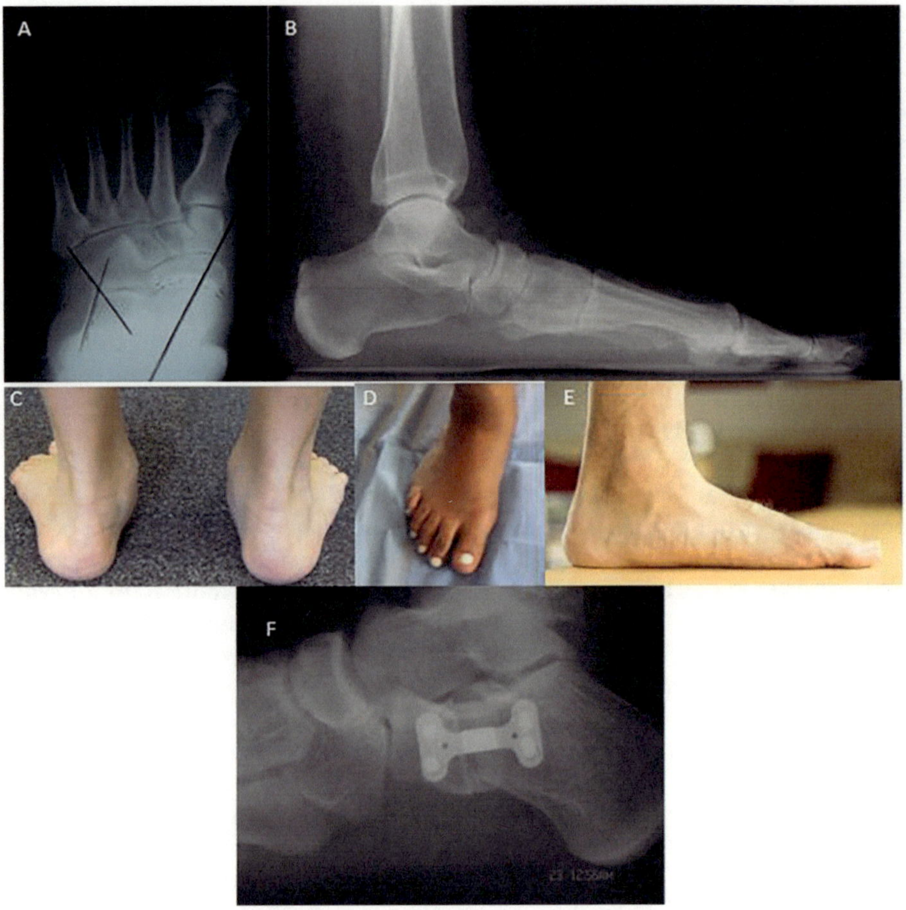

Figure 8.
A: DP view of a transverse (midtarsal type) plane flatfeet; B: lateral view of transverse (midtarsal type) plane flatfeet; C: clinical photograph showing the posterior view of transverse (midtarsal type) plane flatfeet; D: clinical photograph showing the front view of transverse (midtarsal type) plane flatfeet; E: clinical photograph showing the side view of transverse (midtarsal type) plane flatfeet; F: Evans calcaneal osteotomy with screw and plate fixation.

the lateral view (**Figure 8B**) with a mild NC fault (greater than 6 degrees of heel valgus and a near normal Meary's angle). In this case the pronation of the STJ leads to unlocking of the midtarsal joint and forefoot abduction being generated at this level. Arch lowering thus occurs at the first ray and OMTJ "dorsiflexion."

5.2.2 Clinical presentation of the transverse plane flatfoot-midtarsal joint type

When viewing the patient from behind again, (**Figure 8C**) one can see heel valgus of about 8–10 degrees. There is an associated "too-many toes sign" indicating increased forefoot abduction. When viewing the patient from the front no significant talar bulge is noted. The medial malleolus is what appears prominent (**Figure 8D**). This corresponds with the increased talar adduction but internal tibio-fibular rotation as part of closed kinetic chain pronation. Forefoot abduction is noted here as a result of the unlocked CC joint OMTJ. Dorsiflexion also occurs to lower the longitudinal arch laterally and leads to lowering of the medial longitudinal arch (**Figure 8F**).

5.3 Surgical management of transverse flatfoot-midtarsal and subtalar types

To be able to differentiate between the two types clinically, one first places the patient's STJ in a neutral or slightly supinated position. If the forefoot remains locked, then a STJ stabilizing procedure is performed along with a posterior group lengthening. This can be represented by either a posterior calcaneal osteotomy (Koutsogiannis, Gleich-Dwyer) or arthroeresis. The medial column may need a Cotton (opening wedge medical cuneiform osteotomy) or a plantarflexed medial cuneiform osteotomy (Mosca) [12].

If, however when the STJ is placed in a neutral or slightly supinated position, and the forefoot becomes unlocked, then one would address the deformity at the OMTJ level with an Evans opening wedge calcaneal osteotomy (**Figure 8F**) or opening-wedge osteotomy of the cuboid. Similarly, an equinus release may be required as well as a medial column procedure of a Cotton or a PF medial cuneiform osteotomy.

5.3.1 Biomechanics of the transverse plane flatfoot-Kidner foot

When considering a Kidner-type flatfoot one must be aware of the three types of accessory navicular bone. The type I represents the true accessory or sesamoid bone called the os tibiale externum (**Figure 9A**). The second is a so called "pre-hallux" or Gorilloid navicular (**Figure 9B**). It represents a syndesmotic "fibrous" articulation with the main body of the navicular. The third is cornuate navicular which represents an enlarged navicular tuberosity (**Figure 9C**).

In most instances it is the type II accessory navicular that proves to be symptomatic. In this case, the insertion of the tibialis posterior tendon engages primarily the accessory portion. As a result, it becomes functionally weakened. The result is a destabilization of the peritalar complex leading to pronation. The net result is increased talar adduction, plantarflexion and calcaneal eversion. The distal tendinous investments across the midfoot become less effective. With functional alteration of the main insertion of the tibialis posterior tendon and a mechanical advantage to the peroneus brevis is gained. The result is increased forefoot abduction that can be generated at the STJ level but also can evolve about the midtarsal joint (OMTJ). Equinus also can represent a deforming force. Recently fusion or arthrodesis has been performed to stabilize the tibialis posterior tendon function and spring ligament. This was performed on type II navicular conditions [13].

5.3.2 Radiographic evaluation of the transverse plane flatfoot-Kidner foot

In the type I, one can see the presence of an os tibiale externum. In the type II, an associated synchondrosis is present with the main navicular body. The type III has an enlarged cornuate tuberosity. On the DP view (**Figure 9D**), there is an increase in the TC angle. The CA angle in most instances is increased. On the lateral view (**Figure 9E**) there is increased talar plantarflexion and a decrease CI. There is also the presence of a NC break. Meary's angle is decreased due to the inherent degree of heel valgus and equinus.

5.3.3 Clinical presentation of the transverse plane flatfoot-Kidner type

When viewing the patient from behind (**Figure 9F**) one notes an increased amount of heel valgus with 12–14 degrees. There is also the presence of forefoot

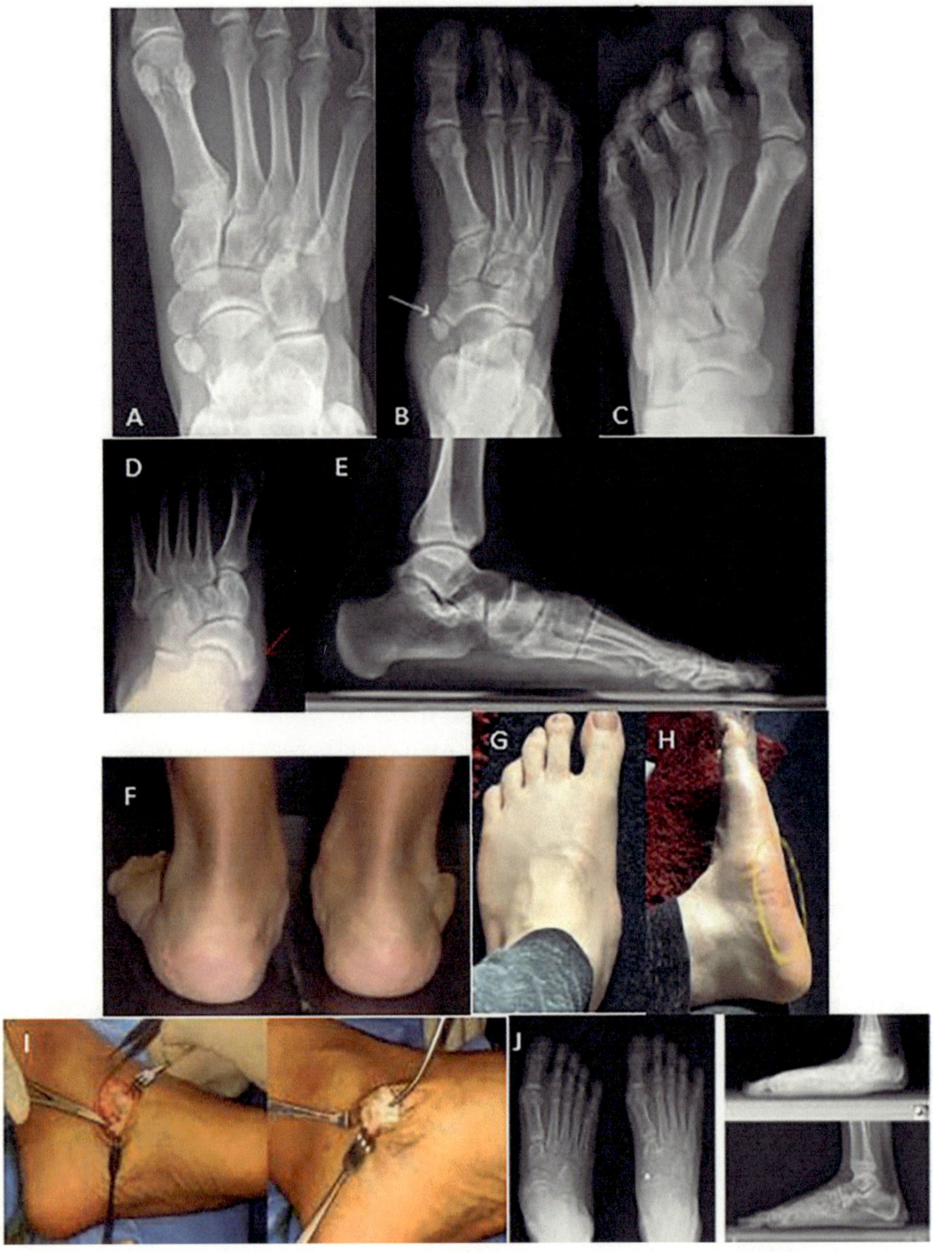

Figure 9.
A: DP view depicting a type I accessory navicular bone; B: DP view depicting a type II Gorilloid navicular bone; C: DP view depicting a type III cornuate navicular bone; D: DP view of a transverse (Kidner type) plane flatfoot; E: lateral view of a transverse (Kidner type) plane flatfoot; F: clinical photograph showing the posterior view of transverse (Kidner type) plane flatfeet; G: clinical photograph showing the dorsal view of transverse (Kidner type) plane flatfoot; H: clinical photograph showing the lateral view of transverse (Kidner type) plane flatfoot; I: Kidner procedure showing removal of navicular tuberosity; J: pre-operative (left) and post-operative radiographs (right).

abduction noted by the "too-many-toes sign." One also notes the increased girth and enlargement due to the enlarged navicular tuberosity. Viewing the patient from the front or dorsal view (**Figure 9G**), one notes increased forefoot abduction and enlarged prominence of the navicular tuberosity. When viewing the patient from the side (**Figure 9H**), one notes weight bearing primarily over the navicular tuberosity.

5.3.4 Surgical management of transverse plane flatfoot-Kidner type

Initial evaluation includes the Silverskold test to determine presence of gastrocnemius or soleus equinus present. Depending, a Bowman or Strayer technique is utilized for gastroc-soleus contracture and a Hoke percutaneous lengthening for gastroc-soleus contracture.

In the case where on the DP view there is an increased TC angle but the CA angle remains normal, a posterior type Koutsogiannis calcaneal osteotomy is performed. If there is also an associated increase in the CA angle, an Evans type opening wedge type osteotomy of the calcaneus is performed. A double calcaneal osteotomy is considered in the presence of more severe signs of instability at the TC and CC joints.

Next step is the performance of Kidner procedure itself. This involves surgical excision and resection of the remaining body parallel to the talus and medial cuneiform (**Figure 9I**). Resection of the navicular body is done at an angled approach. As the resection begins superior it angles medial to lateral when reaching the inferior portion. The result is the tibialis posterior tendon is tensioned with the foot fully supinated at the rearfoot and pronated at the forefoot. This is done with a suture anchor technique. This often will correct the NC fault but in some cases a Cotton opening medial wedge osteotomy or Mosca-type closing wedge osteotomy is needed. The Mosca-type plantarflexory osteotomy does create increased forefoot adduction (**Figure 9J**).

5.4 Biomechanics of the transverse plane flatfoot-Lisfranc type

In this case there has been injury, involving Lisfranc's ligament or degenerative changes of the medial pillar of Lisfranc's joint. This involves the medial (first-met-MC) and central columns (TMT 2, 3). As is known these three joints demonstrate only mono-planar motion. When injury to the deep (plantar) portion of the Lisfranc's ligament occurs, resultant tri-planar instability occurs at the first-met-MC and bi-planar compensation at TMT 2,3. With this instability the first metatarsal dorsiflexes, everts and abducts. This leads to lowering of the arch at the medial cuneiform level and creates a midfoot flatfoot. The central column (TMT 2,3) also dorsiflex and abduct and lower the transverse (Roman) arch. This also serves to shorten the lever arm of the foot which leads to a significant mechanical advantage to the gastrocnemius soleus muscle group and thus equinus contracture. With this pathologic hypermobility pronatory forces are compensated solely at those levels. The clinical result is a midfoot flatfoot with the CORA at the MC joint. Thus, STJ and MTJ compensation will rarely occur, but can in longstanding cases.

5.4.1 Radiographic evaluation of the transverse plane flatfoot-Lisfranc type

On the DP view (**Figure 10A**), one sees shortening (lateral rotation of the first metatarsal on the medial cuneiform). There is a lateral step off of the second and third metatarsals on their respective cuneiforms. Degenerative joint disease occurs dependent on deformity longevity. One notes normal TC and CA angles.

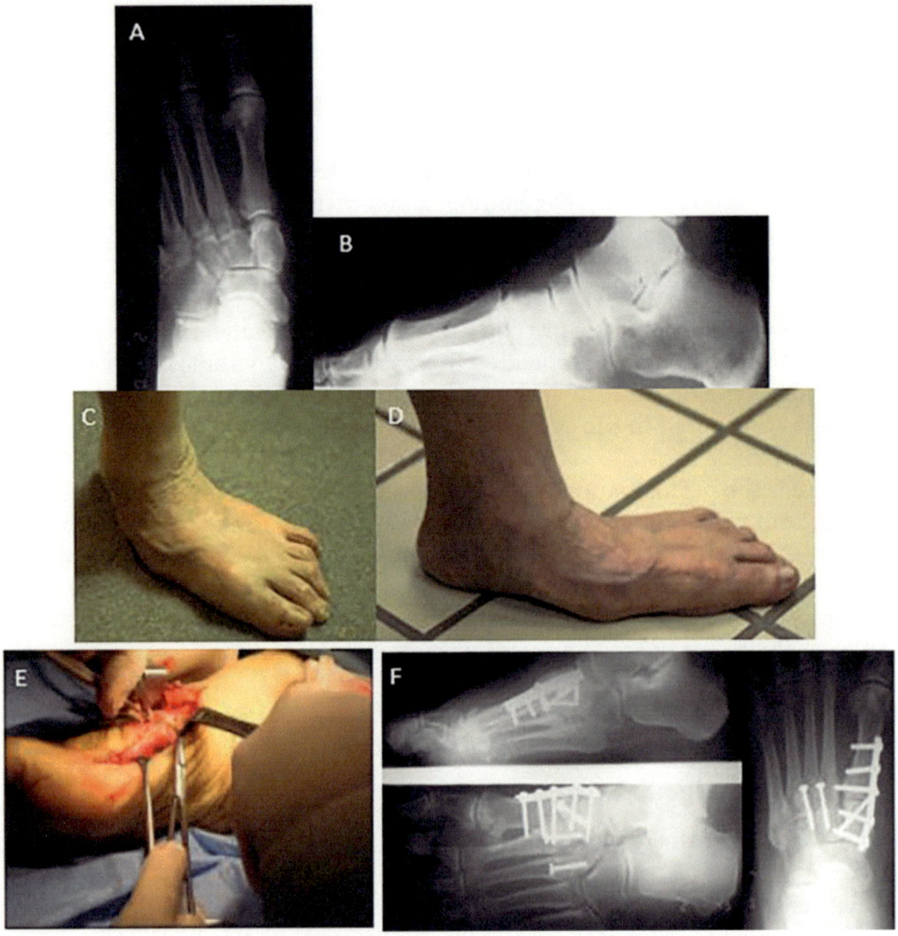

Figure 10.
A: DP view of transverse (Lisfranc's type) plane flatfeet; B: lateral view of transverse (Lisfranc's type) plane flatfeet; C: clinical photograph showing the front view of transverse (Lisfranc type) plane flatfoot; D: clinical photograph showing the side view of transverse (Lisfranc type) plane flatfoot; E: interpositional allograft required as large gap is present upon repositioning of the first metatarsal for surgical management of transverse flatfoot-Lisfranc type; F: surgical management of transverse plane (Lisfranc type) flatfoot.

On the lateral view (**Figure 10B**), one notes a dorsal step off of the first metatarsal base to the MC indicating joint instability. Also, the fifth metatarsal is parallel to the floor indicating increased lateral column instability. The talar declination and CI angle remain normal indicating lack of STJ and MTJ compensation.

5.4.2 Clinical presentation of the transverse plane flatfoot-Lisfranc type

From behind, the calcaneus may show some compensatory eversion, but in most cases, the STJ and MTJ are not involved in compensation.

On a front view (**Figure 10C**), the forefoot is abducted at tarsometatarsal joint with the ankle aligned.

On a side view (**Figure 10D**), the arch is flattened to ground with medial cuneiform weightbearing and loss of transverse arch.

5.4.3 Surgical management of transverse flatfoot-Lisfranc type

The initial approach requires equinus contracture determinant by the Silverskold test. This is effected by the shortened lever arm and most often represents a gastrocnemius contracture. Thus, a Bowman or Strayer-type lengthening is performed.

Next, one must address the instability and if present the degeneration of the medial and central columns. It is critical that the first-met-MC joint be re-established in its plantarflexed, adducted and inverted position. This requires arthrodesis and in some instances due to shortening an interpositional auto or allograft is needed (**Figure 10E**).

The central column (TMT 2, 3) require plantarflexion and adduction to re-establish proper joint alignment by arthrodesis. Care must be performed not to allow shortening or elevation of those respective metatarsals. Any instability or deformity of the lateral column (TMT 4, 5) is addressed by re-alignment and k-wire fixation, no attempt of arthrodesis is performed at this level (**Figure 10F**).

6. Sagittal plane flatfoot deformity

6.1 Biomechanics of the sagittal plane flatfoot deformity

In this deformity centering is about the peritalar complex. The axis in this situation will tilt 45 degrees sagittal, 30 degrees to the frontal and 15 degrees to the transverse planes. The result is a severely maligned talus with significant subluxation at the calcaneus and navicular. This condition has been referred to as an oblique talus. The deformity is semi-flexible. The talus is nearly dislocated at the navicular and subluxed off the STT. Resulting in severe heel valgus with the talar head being weight bearing. There is some amount of translation of the talar articular surface with the navicular. Leading to a mild increase in forefoot abduction noted as an increased CA angle. Also, abhorrence of the TN (LMTJ) axis allows excessive motion in response to the severe heel valgus and equinus.

6.2 Radiographic evaluation of the sagittal plane flatfoot

On the DP view (**Figure 11A**) there is a significant increase in the TC angle. The uncoverage angle can be near 70% or greater. There is an increase in the CA angle leading to increased forefoot abduction.

The axial view (**Figure 11B**) will note hypoplasia of the sustentaculum with the talus subluxed medial and forward. Loss of facet parallelity is present. The anterior and middle facets are not visualized.

On the lateral view (**Figure 11C**) the talus is oblique and an uncharacteristic TN fault is present. The neck of the talus is shortened due to increased compressive intraarticular forces created by the semi flexible, subluxed condition and associated severe equinus. The calcaneal inclination angle (CI) is often negative due to the weight bearing force directed forward and medial at the STT. Equinus force also pulls the calcaneal tuber superiorly. Forefoot supinatus is noted as a piling of the metatarsals due to the longitudinal midtarsal joint abhorrence and alteration. One when viewing the axial and lateral views would consider a STJ coalition.

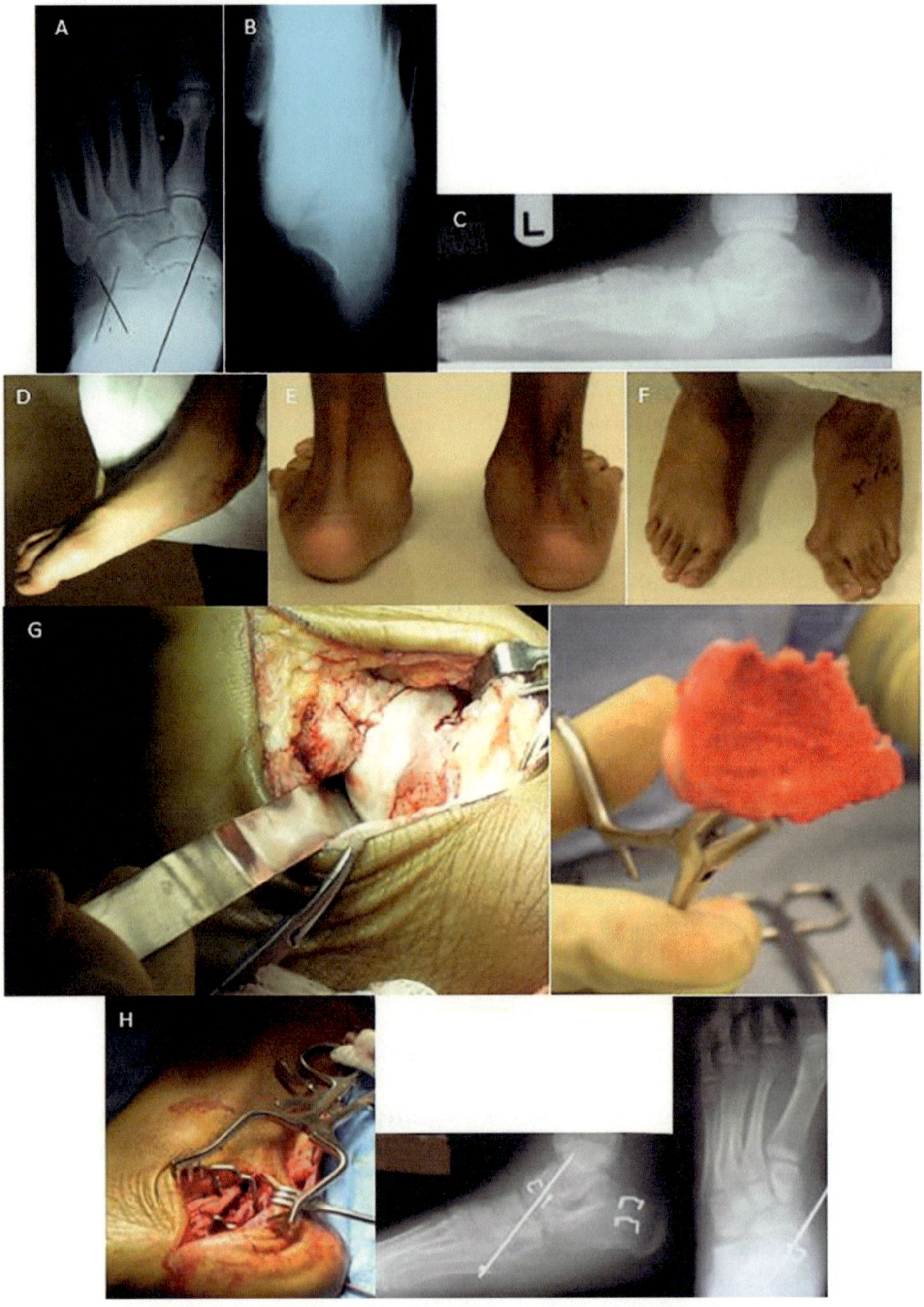

Figure 11.
A: DP radiograph view of a left foot sagittal plane flatfoot; B: axial radiograph view of a sagittal plane flatfoot; C: lateral radiograph view of a left foot sagittal plane flatfoot; D: clinical photograph showing the lateral view of right sagittal plane flatfoot; E: clinical photograph showing the posterior view of sagittal plane flatfeet; F: clinical photograph showing the front view of sagittal plane flatfeet; G: surgical management of a sagittal plane flatfoot depicting sub-capital talar head wedge resection; H: proposed surgical management of a sagittal plane flatfoot with z-plasty of tendoachilles lengthening, Koutsogiannis calcaneal osteotomy.

6.3 Clinical presentation of the sagittal plane flatfoot

When viewing the patient in a non-weight bearing position (**Figure 11D**) the foot appears flattened with loss of the longitudinal arch. This differs from frontal and transverse plane dominated flatfoot deformities which are flexible and the arch appears normal where the longitudinal arch collapses with weight bearing. The lack of flexibility due to TN subluxation allows this clinical condition.

When viewing the patient from behind (**Figure 11E**) one notes severe heel valgus, the plantar heels are not weight bearing secondary to the severe equinus contractures. There is considerable increased girth of the foot due to significant subluxed position of the talus. It appears similar to a patient with a STJ coalition.

One can see when viewing the patient from the front (**Figure 11F**) one can see severe hallux abducto valgus but the forefoot is abducted in the transverse plane. Weight bearing and CORA occur at the talar head level.

6.4 Surgical management of sagittal plane flatfoot deformity

The initial approach is to address the equinus contracture that involves the Achilles tendon. An open z-plasty is required to allow sagittal plane correction of the calcaneus (to increase the calcaneal pitch). A biplane calcaneal osteotomy corrects valgalization and create a vertical heel position. The calcaneal pitch is also corrected.

Due to the fact it is an adolescent or young adult, one needs preserve joint function and avoid arthrodesis if possible. Thus, a talar closing sub capital adductory wedge osteotomy allows correction of the TN fault by shortening the medial column (**Figure 11G**). A Steinmann pin is utilized to correct the compensatory soft tissue contracture of forefoot supinatus by de-rotation around the TN joint. The osteotomy is secured with a staple. One can see by the dissection technique that preservation of the blood supply to the talus is accomplished (**Figure 11H**). It may require lengthening of the tibialis anterior tendon to fully reduce the deformity.

7. Conclusion

In the clinical pictures presented below, the concept of planal dominance via Cardan coupling is presented. Considering primary frontal plane compensation. **Figure 12.1A** demonstrates collapse of the medial longitudinal arch. Clearly the point of weight bearing CORA lies at the navicular and MC articulation. In **Figure 12.1B**, one notes significant calcaneal valgus exceeding 12–16 degrees. In **Figure 12.1C**, one sees the reverse "peek-a-boo" heel sign due to increased heel valgus but also the forefoot is relatively well aligned.

Considering transverse plane dominance we can see four separate modes of compensation. In **Figure 12.2A**, we see STJ compensation with extreme medial talar bulging but the talus not the CORA of weight bearing. A large amount of forefoot abduction at the TN level and a lowered arch with weight bearing at the NC joint. In **Figure 12.2B**, we see the midtarsal joint level, compensation with increased forefoot abduction but prominence medially is the medial malleolus. Arch collapse over the NC joint in **Figure 12.3C**. A Kidner foot with significant forefoot abduction at the midtarsal joint level due to the mechanical imbalance of the peroneus brevis. Again, the NC serves as the weight bearing CORA of the longitudinal arch. **Figure 12.2D**, we have

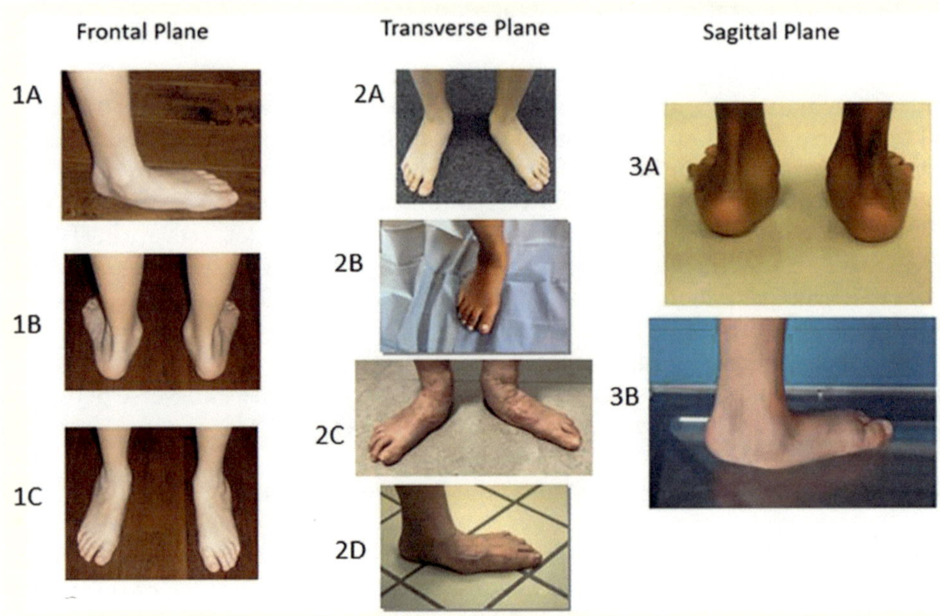

Figure 12.
Summary chart with images depicts the various planal appearances of flat feet.

the "midfoot flatfoot" due to a Lisfranc's medial and central column insufficiency. The weight bearing CORA is at the medial cuneiform itself. Forefoot abduction is at the metatarsal level itself as well as medial and central column of Lisfranc's joint.

In sagittal plane primary compensation one sees from **Figure 12.3A**, from behind, severe heel valgus, the calcaneus not weight bearing due to severe equinus. Significant increase in medial girth is present from the oblique positioning of the talus. On **Figure 12.3B**, clearly the CORA is at the talar head itself where the longitudinal arch appears broken.

Thus not all flatfeet are the same. Axis alteration due to joint morphology determines the major plane of compensation amongst these multiple tri-planar joint.

Conflict of interest

The authors declare no conflict of interest.

Author details

H. John Visser* and Nicole Marie Smith
SSM Health DePaul Hospital Foot and Ankle Surgery Residency, St. Louis, MO, United States

*Address all correspondence to: tsarhjv@aol.com

References

[1] Dowsett JF. Advanced Constructive Geometry. American Branch, New York: Oxford University Press; 1927

[2] Root M, Orien W, Weed J. Biomechanical Evaluation of the Foot. Los Angeles: Clinical Biomechanics Corporation; 1971

[3] Borelli AH, Smith SD. Surgical considerations in the treatment of pes planus. Journal of the American Podiatric Medical Association. 1988;**78**:305

[4] Chambers EF. An operation for the correction of flexible flat feet of adolescents. Western Journal of Surgery, Obstetrics, and Gynecology. 1946;**54**:77-86

[5] Zitzlsperger SMD. The mechanics of the foot based on the concept of the skeleton as a statically indetermined space framework. Clinical Orthopaedics;**16**:47-63

[6] Imsdahl SI, Stender CJ, Cook BK, Pangrazzi G, Patthanacharoenphon C, Sangeorzan BJ, et al. Anteroposterior translational malalignment of ankle arthrodesis alters foot biomechanics in cadaveric gait simulation. Journal of Orthopaedic Research: Official Publication of the Orthopaedic Research Society. 2020;**38**(2):450-458

[7] Prendergast PJ, Huiskes R. The biomechanics of Wolff's law: Recent advances. Irish Journal of Medical Science. 1995;**164**(2):152-154. DOI: 10.1007/BF02973285

[8] Koutsogiannis E. Treatment of mobile flat foot by displacement osteotomy of the calcaneus. Journal of Bone and Joint Surgery. British Volume (London). 1971;**53**:96-100

[9] Vogler H. Subtalar joint blocking operations for pathological pronation syndromes. In: McGlamery ED, editor. Comprehensive Textbook of Foot Surgery. Baltimore: Williams & Wilkins; 1987. pp. 466-482

[10] Smith SD, Ocampo RF. Subtalar arthroresis and associated procedures. Clinics in Podiatric Medicine and Surgery. 1997;**14**(1):87-98

[11] Pisani G. Trattato di chirurgia del piede. Torino: Ediziioni Minerva Medica; 1990

[12] Mosca VS. Principles and Management of Pediatric Foot and Ankle Deformities and Malformations. 1st ed. Philadelphia, PA: Wolters Kluwer/ Lippincott Williams & Wilkins; 2014

[13] Sun N, Chen J, Chen Z, Zeng C, Guo H. Clinical outcomes of fusion in type II accessory naviculars with or without asymptomatic flatfeet. Foot & Ankle International. 2023;**44**(2):139-147. DOI: 10.1177/10711007221140847

Section 4

Causes and Effects of Hindfoot

Chapter 5

Hindfoot Pathologies

Elif Tuğçe Çil

Abstract

Foot pain (FP) is widespread throughout the population, with prevalence estimates ranging from 17 to 30%, while a comprehensive study found that more than one-quarter of people over the age of 45 have regular hindfoot pain (HP). HP has been linked to limitations in daily living activities, poor balance, gait issues, and poor health-related quality of life. According to studies, at least two-thirds of people have moderate functional daily living issues. Aging, female gender, obesity, chronic medical conditions (such as osteoarthritis and diabetes), biomechanical factors (excessive external rotation of the lower extremity, increased pronation of the subtalar joint, plantar flexor weakness, Achilles tendon shortening), and anatomical changes (pes planus, pes cavus) have all been identified as risk factors for HP. People with HP have bone and soft-tissue overload, foot anatomic disorders, and a decreased range of motion (especially ankle dorsiflexion). There are several hindfoot pathologies that can lead to HP. The aim of this study is to overview the pathologies of the hindfoot that cause hindfoot pain.

Keywords: disorder, foot, hindfoot, pain, pathologies

1. Introduction

The hindfoot is the area of the foot located behind the ankle joint, and it is made up of several bones, including the calcaneus (heel bone), talus (ankle bone), and the navicular and cuboid bones [1]. The hindfoot is an important part of the foot and ankle, as it provides support and stability when standing and walking [2]. However, the hindfoot is also susceptible to a wide range of pathologies that can cause pain, swelling, and difficulty moving the foot and ankle [2, 3].

Hindfoot pathologies can be caused by a variety of factors, including overuse, trauma, degeneration, and underlying medical conditions [3]. Some common hindfoot pathologies include posterior tibial tendinopathy, flexor halluces longus tendinopathy, posterior ankle impingement syndrome, heel contusion, calcaneal and talar stress fractures, rheumatoid arthritis of the hindfoot, Paget disease of the hindfoot, osteomyelitis of the calcaneus, and metastatic disease of the foot and ankle [3, 4].

Symptoms of hindfoot pathologies may include pain, swelling, and tenderness in the affected area, as well as difficulty moving the foot and ankle [2, 3]. The condition may also cause deformities or other changes in the appearance of the foot and ankle [4, 5]. Hindfoot sensations occur beneath the ankle and are sometimes mistaken for ankle discomfort [5, 6]. Flat feet and soreness are caused by issues such as posterior tibial tendon insufficiency. On the inside or outside of hindfoot, pain might occur [6].

Chronic conditions	Overuse tendon conditions	Traumatic conditions	Medical conditions
Plantar fasciitis	Peroneal tendon injury	Posterior ankle impingement syndrome	Rheumatologic disease
Tarsal tünel syndrome	Posterior tibial tendinopathy	Heel contusion	Paget disease
Achilles tendinopathy & hallung deformity	Flexor hallucis longus tendinopathy	Calcaneal & talar stress fractures	Osteomyelitis of calcaneus
Sinüs tarsi syndrome			Sickle cell disease
Piezogenic papules			Gout
Subtalar arthritis			Metastatic disease

Table 1.
Categorization of hindfoot pathologies.

This also causes symptoms of weakness and instability around the ankle and hindfoot [2, 3]. Stress fractures, ankle instability, and peroneal tendonitis can all be caused by having a high-arch foot [4, 5]. Arthritis can also affect the hindfoot, causing dull discomfort, stiffness, and deformity later on. Swelling or edema in the hindfoot area may indicate inflammatory or joint soft-tissue processes [6]. It is important to seek medical treatment for hindfoot pathologies to prevent the condition from worsening and to maintain good function of the foot and ankle. Early diagnosis and treatment can help to alleviate symptoms and prevent further damage to the foot and ankle.

The pathologies that present with HP are presented in **Table 1**.

2. Hindfoot pathologies

2.1 Chronic conditions

2.1.1 Plantar fasciitis (PF)

The most common cause of plantar heel pain is plantar fasciitis, which is a chronic degenerative irritation of the plantar fascia origin at the medial calcaneal tuberosity as well as surrounding perifascial structures such as the plantar aponeurosis of the foot [7]. This condition is primarily a degenerative process [7, 8]. Histologic samples from PF patients undergoing plantar fascia surgery demonstrate myxoid degeneration with fragmentation, collagen disarray, granulation tissue, micro-tears, bone marrow vascular ectasia, and lack of traditional inflammation [8, 9]. Additionally, ultrasound assessment often finds calcifications, tears, thickening, and plantar fascia heterogeneity. These changes, commonly seen on ultrasound, induce a non-inflammatory condition and dysfunctional vasculature. According to these findings, the condition is a degenerative fasciosis without inflammation, not fasciitis. That is why plantar fasciopathy is a more accurate definer. Although the diagnosis includes the portion "itis," the condition is characterized by a lack of inflammatory cells [8, 9].

Although the decisive incidence and prevalence of PF by age are unclear, estimations show that it affects roughly 10% of the general public, with 83% of these patients being active working individuals aged 25–65 [10]. Additionally, it is common in athletic and sedentary populations and associated with a diversity of sports but is primarily reported in elite and recreational runners with 5–10% incidence [7, 10].

The reason for PF is multifactorial, but most cases are due to overuse stress. A heel spur may be found in some cases, but it is not a causative factor. It often takes place in middle-aged (40–60 years) women and is vast in military servicemen, long-distance runners (repetitive strain), and obese people (BMI >27 kg/m^2) [10, 11]. Pes planus, pes cavus, limited ankle DF, and excessive pronation or supination are all predisposing factors. The gastro-soleus and other posterior leg muscles are frequently observed to be tight. Tight muscles can alter typical motion biomechanics. Weight-bearing, age, leg length asymmetry, heel pad atrophy, vocations requiring extended standing, and low-heeled shoes with solid bottoms or tightly fitting shoes are additional risk factors [9–11].

Patients will generally present with low-medial heel progressive pain. In more complicated situations, the pain might radiate proximally. The pain is commonly described as severe and worse with the first few steps in the morning by patients. Long durations of standing or sitting will further aggravate the discomfort. The pain usually subsides after ambulation or the start of athletic activity but often returns later in the day [11, 12]. It may be replicated in most cases by palpating the plantar medial calcaneal tubercle and passive DF of the toes and foot. The windlass test refers to the passive DF of the first metatarsophalangeal joint (positive) [7, 11]. Second, the causative factors may contain a tight AT and pes cavus or planus. That is why assessing a patient's gait may be beneficial [10, 11]. Stress fractures, fat pad contusion or atrophy, and nerve entrapments such as tarsal tunnel syndrome should all be examined in the differential diagnosis of PF [7]. In most cases, clinical diagnosis and imaging are not required [8]. If there is another indication of other injuries or if the patient fails, it may be essential to obtain X-rays or an ultrasound evaluation. Soft-tissue calcifications or heel spurs on the inferior surface of the heel may be seen on X-rays or ultrasonic assessment. The plantar fascia may seem thickened and swollen on ultrasound. Ultrasound findings consistent with PF contain plantar fascia thickness greater than 4.0 mm. If the patient does not respond to conservative therapy after more prolonged periods, then MRI may be considered to assess for fascial tears, stress fractures, or osteochondral defects. Additionally, MRI can demonstrate increased plantar fascia thickness and signal intensity. For evaluating and distinguishing PF, ultrasonography is a cost-effective, precise, and dependable alternative to MRI. Plain radiography can detect bone abnormalities, and lateral heel radiographs can reveal a heel spur. Even though people with chronic HP are more likely to have a spur, it can remain after symptoms resolve [7, 11, 13].

Most cases are managed non-surgically (90%), but the recurrence of pain is an obstruction. An inter-professional approach is necessary because there is no single treatment for everyone. Even when a treatment option works, symptoms frequently take weeks or months to subside [10–12]. It is important to note that surgery for PF is usually only recommended for patients who have not responded to other forms of treatment and are experiencing severe, chronic pain. Plantar fasciitis can be treated surgically using a variety of techniques. These are some examples: plantar fascia release, calcaneal spur excision, tenotomy, and neurectomy. It should be noted that surgery for plantar fasciitis is usually only indicated for people who have not responded to other treatment options.

It is also worth noting that surgery carries risks and is not always successful in relieving pain. It is important to carefully consider all treatment options and discuss the risks and benefits with a healthcare provider before deciding on surgery.

2.1.2 Tarsal tünel syndrome

Tarsal tunnel syndrome is a condition that involves compression of the posterior tibial nerve, which runs through the tarsal tunnel in the hindfoot. The tarsal tunnel is a narrow passageway in the ankle that is formed by bones, ligaments, and tendons. The posterior tibial nerve passes through this tunnel to provide sensation to the foot and toes [14].

Symptoms of tarsal tunnel syndrome may include:

- Pain in the foot, ankle, or toes
- Numbness or tingling in the foot and toes
- Burning or aching sensation in the foot and toes
- Difficulty in the foot or toe mobility

Tarsal tunnel syndrome is often caused by overuse, injury, or other conditions that put pressure on the posterior tibial nerve. It can also be caused by structural abnormalities in the foot, such as flat feet or high arches [15].

Treatment for tarsal tunnel syndrome may include rest, ice, physical therapy, stretches, and over-the-counter or prescription pain medication. In some cases, a splint or brace may be used to support the foot and reduce pressure on the nerve. Surgery may be necessary if other treatments are not effective [14, 15]. Tarsal tunnel syndrome is usually treated conservatively; however, in some cases, surgery (tarsal tunnel release, decompression surgery, nerve decompression) may be necessary to relieve the pressure on the tibial nerve.

2.1.3 Achilles tendinopathy (AT) & Haglund deformity

Tendinopathy is the degeneration or inability to heal the tendon due to recurrent stress without proper recuperation. AT is a widespread overuse injury, resulting from excessive compression or triceps surae mechanical loading [16]. It divides into mid-portion (non-insertional) and insertional tendinopathy. Discomfort at 2–6 cm from the calcaneal insertion and insertional pain at the Achilles tendon insertion make up the mid-portion. AT is a clinical diagnostic that occurs when a patient has localized discomfort, Achilles tendon edema, and loss of function. In terms of pain localization, Achilles tendon injuries are divided into three categories: midportion tendinopathy (55–65% of injuries), insertional tendinopathy (20–25%), and proximal musculotendinous junction injuries (9–25%) [16–18]. On the other hand, patients have discomfort at the insertion and midportion simultaneously, with around 30% experiencing bilateral pain. Tendinopathy is also marked by increased tissue thickness (tendinosis), a lack of typical collagen, an increase in proteoglycans, and a general breakdown in tissue structure [16, 18]. In both asymptomatic and symptomatic tendons, these structural alterations increase cross-sectional area, reduce tendon stiffness, and modify viscoelastic properties. Furthermore, tendon alteration (tendinosis) is commonly accompanied by other disorders, such as the spread of intratendinous calcifications, bone abnormalities, and the retrocalcaneal bursa in the insertional one [16, 17].

The risk of developing AT is assumed to be multifaceted, with intrinsic and extrinsic variables contributing to either a reduction in load tolerance or a change in movement-pattern stress on the tendon. Reduced PF strength, hip neuromuscular control problems, abnormal DF and subtalar-joint ROM, increased foot pronation, and body weight are all intrinsic risk factors that can be determined. Aside from family history, systemic illness and genetic variations have also been identified as inherent risk factors [17, 19]. Tendinopathy and tendon rupture have been connected to fluoroquinolone antibiotics, with symptoms appearing 8 days after therapy begins. Sport involvement, footwear, surface, training-load mistakes (such as an immediate increase in training length or intensity, a reduction in recovery time), and ambient variables have all been linked to AT development because of a lack of data [18, 19].

The primary symptoms are pain and decreased function. Patients generally explain a gradual onset of symptoms with morning stiffness or after prolonged sitting, pain with palpation and activity (jumping or running), and damages in strength or performance. Activity pain can vary in terms of severity. The initial symptom can merge with the start of the activity. It is relatively unusual for an athlete to have poor athletic performance (e.g., decreased jogging time or jump performance) before experiencing discomfort during the activity. Athletes who overlook small indications may feel discomfort during and after exertion and experience a decline in performance. It is crucial to note that in the absence of loading, people with AT typically experience no discomfort [18, 20].

The subjective report of discomfort and pain with tendon palpation is a reliable and valid diagnostic for AT. Palpation of pain can help distinguish between insertional-midportion damage and a diagnosis. For example, if palpating the anterior tendon causes more discomfort than the tendon, os trigonum syndrome or posterior ankle impingement may be a more likely diagnosis. Acute AT rupture, accessory soleus, systemic inflammatory illness, sural nerve, and fat-pad irritation are more factors to consider in posterior ankle discomfort [16, 18, 19]. Additionally, diagnostic tests like the Royal London Hospital test and the arc sign may be performed to confirm AT [16, 20]. Patient-reported pain and symptoms have traditionally been used to determine the severity of the condition.

Nevertheless, patients also have increased fear of movement, or kinesiophobia; impaired lower extremity function; altered tendon structure; and decreased muscle performance. The patient's overall condition rating, participation, pain on loading or activity or over a certain length of time, function, psychological aspects, physical function capacity, disability, and quality of life are all factors that contribute to a consensus [16, 17]. Patients with AT have varying degrees of impairment and symptoms in each domain. Each component of tendon health must be assessed for diagnostic progress, patient objectives and expectations, and athlete return-to-sport decisions. In addition, structural changes might occur without causing any symptoms. Other patients may experience symptoms and functional impairments with no structural change. Furthermore, complete symptomatic healing does not guarantee complete functional recovery. As a result, the effective reinjury rates (27–44%) for AT may be due to merely using symptom resolution as a recovery guide without confirming tendon health [17–19].

Pathophysiology related to AT is frequently determined by imaging. Existence of osteophyte and enthesophyte formation, Haglund deformity, and intratendinous calcifications, evaluation may all be determined with lateral weight-bearing radiographs of the foot. The form and lucency of the Kager triangle on a radiograph may also be utilized to determine whether or not a patient has retrocalcaneal bursitis. Ultrasound and MRI may be used to evaluate soft-tissue (bursitis, neovascularization, paratendinitis, tendon degeneration) as well as bony (intratendinous calcification, enthesophytes) changes [19, 20].

Haglund deformity is a bony enlargement at the back of the heel that can cause pain and discomfort when walking or wearing certain types of shoes. It is also known as "pump bump" because it is often caused by the irritation and pressure that can occur when wearing high-heeled pumps. The deformity is caused by a combination of genetics and the way that a person walks. It is more common in people who have high arches and who walk with a gait that places extra stress on the heels. It can also be caused by inflammation of the bursa, a small fluid-filled sac that acts as a cushion between the heel bone and the Achilles tendon. Symptoms of Haglund deformity include pain and swelling at the back of the heel, redness and warmth in the affected area, and difficulty wearing certain types of shoes. Treatment may include wearing shoes with a low heel or wide toe box, using padding or inserts in the shoes, and taking over-the-counter pain medications. In severe cases, surgery may be necessary to remove the bony growth and relieve pressure on the heel.

Debridement: This procedure involves removing damaged tissue from the Achilles tendon to reduce inflammation and pain.

Tenotomy: This procedure involves cutting the Achilles tendon to release tension and alleviate pain.

Haglund deformity excision: This procedure involves removing the bony growth on the back of the heel.

It is important to note that surgery for AT and Haglund deformity is usually only recommended for patients who have not responded to other forms of treatment and are experiencing severe, chronic pain [21, 22].

2.1.4 Sinüs tarsi syndrome

Sinus tarsi syndrome is a condition that affects the sinus tarsi, a small cavity located in the ankle joint. It is characterized by pain, swelling, and instability in the ankle and can be caused by a variety of factors, including injury, arthritis, and structural abnormalities in the foot [23].

The sinus tarsi is a small, triangular-shaped space located between the talus (ankle bone) and the calcaneus (heel bone). It is filled with a fibrous tissue called the interosseous talocalcaneal ligament, which helps to stabilize the ankle joint and absorb shock during movement [3].

Sinus tarsi syndrome is often caused by trauma to the ankle, such as a sprain or fracture. It can also be caused by structural abnormalities in the foot, such as flat feet or high arches, which can put extra strain on the ligaments and joints of the ankle. Arthritis, particularly osteoarthritis, can also lead to sinus tarsi syndrome, as the degenerative changes in the joint can cause pain and instability [24].

Symptoms of sinus tarsi syndrome can include pain, swelling, and instability in the ankle, as well as difficulty walking or standing on the affected foot. The pain is typically worse when the foot is rotated outward or when weight is placed on the outer edge of the foot [24, 25].

Treatment for sinus tarsi syndrome may include rest, ice, and physical therapy to help strengthen the muscles and ligaments in the ankle. In severe cases, surgery may be necessary to repair any damage to the sinus tarsi or surrounding structures. Sinus tarsi decompression, sinus tarsi stabilization, or sinus tarsi fusion surgical procedures may be necessary to relieve pain and improve stability [24, 25].

2.1.5 Piezogenic papules

Piezogenic papules are small, painless bumps that typically appear on the heels of the feet. They are caused by the herniation of fat through the fascia, a connective tissue layer that surrounds the muscles [26].

Piezogenic papules are often seen in people who are overweight or obese, as excess body fat can put extra pressure on the fascia and cause the fat to protrude through the tissue. They are also more common in people who engage in activities that involve a lot of running or jumping, as the impact on the heels can cause the fat to herniate [27].

Piezogenic papules are typically harmless and do not cause any symptoms. They may be cosmetically unpleasant for some people, but they do not require treatment. However, if you are experiencing pain or discomfort in your heels, it is important to speak with a healthcare provider to determine the cause and discuss treatment options. In some cases, piezogenic papules may be a sign of underlying issues with the feet, such as flat feet or high arches, which can lead to discomfort and other problems if left untreated [26, 27]. There is no specific treatment for piezogenic papules, and they often resolve on their own over time. In some cases, however, people may choose to have them removed surgically. The surgical procedure used to remove piezogenic papules is called a fat-pad excision. During this procedure, a small incision is made in the skin over the papule, and the protruding fat is removed. The incision is then closed with sutures. It is important to note that surgery for piezogenic papules is usually only recommended for patients who are bothered by the appearance of the papules and have not responded to other forms of treatment.

2.1.6 Subtalar arthritis

Subtalar arthritis is a type of arthritis that affects the subtalar joint, which is a small joint located between the talus (ankle bone) and the calcaneus (heel bone). This joint is responsible for allowing the foot to move and rotate, and it plays an important role in the normal function of the foot and ankle [28].

Subtalar arthritis is characterized by inflammation and degeneration of the subtalar joint. It can be caused by a variety of factors, including injury, overuse, or wear and tear on the joint. Symptoms of subtalar arthritis may include pain, swelling, stiffness, and limited range of motion in the foot and ankle [29].

Treatment for subtalar arthritis may include a combination of conservative measures such as rest, ice, physical therapy, and medications to reduce pain and inflammation. In more severe cases, surgery (arthrodesis, osteotomy, arthroplasty) may be necessary to repair or reconstruct the joint. It is important to seek medical treatment for subtalar arthritis to prevent the condition from worsening and to maintain good function of the foot and ankle. Early diagnosis and treatment can help to alleviate symptoms and prevent further damage to the joint [28, 29].

2.2 Overuse tendon conditions

2.2.1 Peroneal tendon injury

Peroneal tendon injuries are injuries to the tendons in the lower leg that are responsible for moving and stabilizing the ankle and foot. The peroneal tendons are located on the outside of the lower leg, just behind the bone on the outside of the ankle (the fibula). There are two main peroneal tendons: the peroneus longus and the peroneus brevis. These tendons are responsible for moving the foot and ankle outward (everting) and helping the ankle stabilize [30].

Peroneal tendon injuries can occur due to a variety of causes, including overuse, sudden trauma, or degeneration of the tendons. Symptoms of a peroneal tendon injury may include pain, swelling, and difficulty moving the foot and ankle. In severe cases, the tendons may become partially or completely torn, which can lead to instability of the ankle and foot [31].

Treatment for a peroneal tendon injury may include rest, physical therapy, and medications to reduce pain and inflammation. In severe cases, surgery, which includes tendoscopy, tendon repair, and tendon reconstruction, may be necessary to repair or reconstruct the damaged tendons. It is important to seek medical treatment for a peroneal tendon injury to prevent the condition from worsening and to maintain good function of the foot and ankle. Early diagnosis and treatment can help to alleviate symptoms and prevent further damage to the tendons [30, 31].

2.2.2 Posterior tibial tendinopathy

Posterior tibial tendinopathy is a condition that affects the posterior tibial tendon, which is a large tendon located in the lower leg that is responsible for supporting the arch of the foot and helping the ankle stabilize. The posterior tibial tendon runs from the back of the tibia (shin bone) and attaches to the bones of the foot. It is an important part of the "arch support" system of the foot, and it helps to maintain proper alignment and stability of the ankle and foot when standing and walking [32].

Posterior tibial tendinopathy is a condition that occurs when the posterior tibial tendon becomes inflamed or damaged. It can be caused by overuse, injury, or degeneration of the tendon. Symptoms of posterior tibial tendinopathy may include pain, swelling, and difficulty moving the foot and ankle. The condition can lead to instability of the ankle and foot, and it may cause the arch of the foot to collapse, leading to a condition called "flatfoot" [33].

Treatment for posterior tibial tendinopathy may include rest, physical therapy, and medications to reduce pain and inflammation. In severe cases, surgery may be necessary to repair or reconstruct the damaged tendon. These surgical procedures that can be used to treat posterior tibial tendinopathy include: tendoscopy, tendon repair, and tendon reconstruction. It is important to seek medical treatment for posterior tibial tendinopathy to prevent the condition from worsening and to maintain good function of the foot and ankle. Early diagnosis and therapy can assist in relieving symptoms and avoiding further tendon damage [32, 33].

2.2.3 Flexor hallucis longus tendinopathy

Flexor hallucis longus (FHL) tendinopathy is a condition that affects the flexor hallucis longus tendon, which is a long, thin tendon located in the lower leg. The flexor hallucis longus tendon runs from the back of the tibia (shin bone) down to the bones of the foot, and it is responsible for flexing (bending) the big toe. The tendon also helps to stabilize the foot and ankle when standing and walking [34].

FHL tendinopathy is a condition that occurs when the flexor hallucis longus tendon becomes inflamed or damaged. It can be caused by overuse, injury, or degeneration of the tendon. Symptoms of FHL tendinopathy may include pain, swelling, and difficulty moving the big toe and foot. The condition can lead to instability of the ankle and foot, and it may cause problems with balance and gait [33, 34].

Treatment for FHL tendinopathy may include rest, physical therapy, and medications to reduce pain and inflammation. Early diagnosis and treatment can help to alleviate symptoms and prevent further damage to the tendon. It is important to point out that surgery for flexor hallucis longus tendinopathy (tendoscopy, tendon repair, tendon reconstruction) is often reserved for patients who have failed to respond to various types of treatment and are experiencing significant, chronic pain or impairment. Before deciding on surgery, it is critical to carefully explore all treatment choices and discuss the risks and benefits with a healthcare expert [23, 33].

2.3 Traumatic conditions

2.3.1 Posterior ankle impingement syndrome

Posterior ankle impingement syndrome is a condition that affects the back of the ankle and is characterized by pain and inflammation in the soft tissues and bones of the ankle. It is often caused by repetitive stress or overuse of the ankle, and it can also be caused by trauma or injury to the ankle. There are two main types of posterior ankle impingement syndrome: soft-tissue impingement and bone impingement. Soft-tissue impingement occurs when the tendons, ligaments, or muscles at the back of the ankle become inflamed or pinched, causing pain and discomfort. Bone impingement occurs when the bones of the ankle rub against each other or become stuck, causing pain and limited range of motion in the ankle [35, 36].

Symptoms of posterior ankle impingement syndrome may include pain and swelling at the back of the ankle, difficulty moving the ankle, and limited range of motion. The condition may also cause difficulty with activities that involve flexing or pointing the foot, such as walking or running [37].

Treatment for posterior ankle impingement syndrome may include rest, ice, physical therapy, and medications to reduce pain and inflammation. In severe cases, surgery may be necessary to remove any bone spurs or repair damaged tendons or ligaments. There are various surgical options, including debridement, tenotomy, osteophyte removal, and ankle fusion. These surgical techniques may be required to reduce discomfort and improve function. It is important to seek medical treatment for posterior ankle impingement syndrome to prevent the condition from worsening and to maintain good function of the ankle. Early detection and management can help relieve the pain and avoid additional ankle damage [35–37].

2.3.2 Heel contusion

A heel contusion is a type of injury that occurs when the heel bone (calcaneus) is struck or compressed, resulting in pain, swelling, and bruising. Heel contusions are often caused by falls, accidents, or impacts to the heel, such as when landing on the heel after a jump. Symptoms of a heel contusion may include pain and swelling at the site of the injury, difficulty walking or bearing weight on the foot, and bruising or discoloration of the skin around the heel. In severe cases, a heel contusion may cause a fracture or crack in the heel bone, which can lead to additional symptoms such as deformity or instability of the foot [38].

Rest, ice, and elevation of the foot are common treatments for a heel contusion to minimize swelling and inflammation. Over-the-counter pain medications may also be used to help alleviate discomfort. In severe cases, a heel contusion may require more advanced treatment, such as immobilization with a cast or crutches, or surgery to repair any fractures or cracks in the heel bone. Surgery may be necessary if the injury has caused significant damage to the bones, tendons, or other structures in the heel. Debridement, tenotomy, and fracture repair surgical methods can be used for a heel contusion. It is crucial to remember that surgery for a heel contusion is usually indicated only for individuals who have not responded to other forms of treatment and are suffering from significant, chronic pain or impairment [23].

2.3.3 Calcaneal and talar stress fractures

Calcaneal (heel bone) and talar (ankle bone) stress fractures are small cracks or fractures that occur in the bones of the foot as a result of repetitive stress or overuse. Stress fractures are a common injury among athletes, particularly those who engage in high-impact activities such as running or jumping [39].

Symptoms of calcaneal or talar stress fractures may include pain, swelling, and tenderness at the site of the fracture, as well as difficulty bearing weight on the affected foot. The pain may be worse with activity and may improve with rest. Stress fractures can also cause changes in the way a person walks or moves, as they try to avoid putting pressure on the affected foot [23].

Treatment for calcaneal or talar stress fractures typically involves rest, ice, and elevation of the foot to reduce swelling and inflammation. Non-weight-bearing activities, such as swimming or biking, may be recommended to allow the bone to heal. In severe cases, a cast or crutches may be necessary to fully immobilize the foot and allow the fracture to heal. It is important to prevent the injury from worsening and to ensure proper healing and recovery. Conservative treatment for calcaneal and talar stress fractures includes rest, physical therapy, and medicines. However, in some circumstances, surgery, including fracture repair, bone grafting, and bone fusion, may be required to heal the fractured bone [23, 39].

2.4 Medical conditions

2.4.1 Rheumatoid arthritis of the hindfoot

Rheumatoid arthritis (RA) is a chronic autoimmune disorder that causes inflammation in the joints. It can affect any joint in the body, including the hindfoot (the area of the foot behind the ankle joint). RA of the hindfoot can cause pain, swelling, stiffness, and deformity of the foot and ankle [40].

The hindfoot is made up of several bones, including the calcaneus (heel bone), talus (ankle bone), and the navicular and cuboid bones. These bones are connected by joints, and in people with RA, these joints can become inflamed and damaged. This can lead to a range of symptoms, including pain, stiffness, and difficulty moving the foot and ankle. RA of the hindfoot may also cause the foot to become misshapen or deformed, leading to problems with balance and gait [41].

Treatment for RA of the hindfoot typically involves a combination of medications and lifestyle changes to reduce inflammation and manage pain. Medications such as nonsteroidal anti-inflammatory drugs (NSAIDs) and disease-modifying antirheumatic drugs (DMARDs) may be used to reduce inflammation and slow the progression of the disease. Physical therapy and other rehabilitation techniques may also be recommended to help improve mobility and function of the foot and ankle. However, in severe cases, joint fusion, joint replacement, and osteotomy surgical procedures may be necessary to repair or reconstruct damaged joints. It is important to seek medical treatment for RA of the hindfoot to prevent the condition from worsening and to maintain good function of the foot and ankle [23, 40, 41].

2.4.2 Paget disease

Paget disease is a chronic bone disorder that causes abnormal bone growth and weakening of the bone. It can affect any bone in the body, including the bones of the hindfoot (the area of the foot behind the ankle joint). In people with Paget disease of the hindfoot, the bones may become thickened, enlarged, and weakened, leading to a range of symptoms, including pain, swelling, and deformity of the foot and ankle. The condition may also cause problems with balance and gait [23, 42].

Treatment for Paget disease of the hindfoot may involve a combination of medications and lifestyle changes to slow the progression of the disease and manage symptoms. Medications such as bisphosphonates and calcitonin may be used to reduce bone resorption and slow the rate of bone growth. Physical therapy and other rehabilitation techniques may also be recommended to help improve mobility and function of the foot and ankle. Paget disease is typically treated with drugs that delay the disease's course and alleviate bone discomfort. However, surgery may be required in some cases to repair abnormalities or support weakening bones. Paget disease can be treated by using a variety of surgical methods (osteotomy, bone grafting, or joint replacement for repairing or reconstructing damaged bones). Treatment as soon as possible can help to ease symptoms and avoid additional bone loss [42].

2.4.3 Osteomyelitis of calcaneus

Osteomyelitis is an infection of the bone that can affect any bone in the body, including the calcaneus (heel bone). Osteomyelitis of the calcaneus is a serious condition that can cause pain, swelling, and difficulty moving the foot and ankle. It can also lead to bone deformities and other complications if left untreated. It is usually caused by bacteria entering the bone through an open wound or a surgical incision. It can also occur as a result of a blood infection (septicemia) that spreads to the bone. Symptoms of osteomyelitis of the calcaneus may include fever, chills, redness and swelling at the site of the infection, and severe pain. The condition may also cause difficulty walking or bearing weight on the affected foot [43].

Treatment for osteomyelitis of the calcaneus typically involves a combination of antibiotics to kill the infection and surgery, which contains debridement, bone grafting, and amputation procedures, to remove any infected or damaged bone tissue. In severe cases, hospitalization may be necessary to monitor the infection and manage the patient's symptoms. Rehabilitation and physical therapy may also be recommended to help improve mobility and function of the foot and ankle. It is important to get early diagnosis and treatment to prevent the infection from spreading and to ensure proper healing, recovery, and prevention of further complications [44].

2.4.4 Sickle cell disease

Sickle cell disease is a group of inherited blood disorders that affect the production of red blood cells. People with sickle cell disease produce abnormal red blood cells that are shaped like crescent moons (or "sickles") instead of the normal round shape.

These abnormal red blood cells are more fragile and prone to breaking down, which can lead to a range of symptoms and complications. It is caused by a genetic mutation that affects the production of the protein hemoglobin, which carries oxygen in the blood. People with sickle cell disease have abnormal hemoglobin in their red blood cells, which causes them to be misshapen and brittle. As a result, the red blood cells are unable to carry oxygen effectively to the body's tissues, leading to a range of symptoms and complications [45].

Symptoms of sickle cell disease may include anemia (low red blood cell count), fatigue, shortness of breath, and repeated infections. The condition may also cause pain crises, which are episodes of severe pain that can occur in any part of the body. People with sickle cell disease may also have an increased risk of developing other health problems, such as stroke, kidney disease, and vision loss [23, 44].

Treatment for sickle cell disease typically involves a combination of medications, blood transfusions, and other supportive care to manage symptoms and prevent complications. There is no cure for sickle cell disease, but with proper treatment and management, people with the condition can lead full and active lives. The specific surgical procedures used to treat sickle cell disease will depend on the specific complications and individual needs of the patient. Some common surgical procedures used in the treatment of sickle cell disease include: splenectomy, vaso-occlusive crisis management, and bone marrow transplant. It is important to note that surgery for sickle cell disease is usually only recommended for patients who experience severe, chronic complications or who have not responded to other forms of treatment. It is also critical to seek medical treatment and adhere to a treatment plan in order to avoid significant problems and retain good health [46].

2.4.5 Gout

Gout is a type of arthritis that causes inflammation and pain in the joints, most commonly the joints of the feet and ankles. It is caused by the buildup of uric acid crystals in the joints, which leads to inflammation and pain. Gout is characterized by sudden, severe attacks of pain and inflammation in the affected joints. The most common symptoms of gout include redness, warmth, and swelling in the affected joint, as well as intense pain and tenderness. The attacks of gout can last for a few days to a few weeks, and they may occur repeatedly over time. It is more common in men than in women, and it is more likely to occur in people who are overweight, have high blood pressure, or have a family history of gout. It can also be caused by certain medications, alcohol use, and other medical conditions [47, 48].

Treatment for gout may include medications to reduce inflammation and pain, as well as lifestyle changes to help prevent future attacks. These may include changes to diet (such as reducing intake of foods high in purines, which can increase uric acid levels), weight loss, and avoiding triggers such as alcohol and certain medications. In severe cases, surgery may be necessary to remove the uric acid crystals from the affected joints. There are several surgical procedures that may be used to treat gout. These include: debridement, joint fusion, and joint replacement. It is important to carefully consider all treatment options and discuss the risks and benefits with a healthcare provider before deciding on surgery. Getting medical treatment for gout to prevent the condition from worsening and to maintain good function of the joints is important [47].

2.4.6 Metastatic disease

Metastatic disease of the foot and ankle is a type of cancer that occurs when cancer cells from another part of the body spread (metastasize) to the bones of the foot and ankle. This can lead to pain, swelling, and other symptoms in the affected area. It is most commonly caused by breast, lung, or prostate cancer, but it can also occur as a result of other types of cancer [23, 49]. Symptoms of metastatic disease of the foot and ankle may include pain, swelling, and tenderness in the affected area, as well as difficulty moving the foot and ankle. The condition may also cause deformities or other changes in the appearance of the foot and ankle [49].

Treatment for metastatic disease of the foot and ankle depends on the type and stage of cancer, as well as the overall health of the patient. Options may include surgery to remove the affected bone, chemotherapy or radiation therapy to kill the cancer cells, or a combination of these treatments. Pain management and rehabilitation may also be necessary to help alleviate symptoms and improve mobility and function of the foot and ankle. The specific surgical procedure used to treat metastatic disease will depend on the location and size of the metastases, as well as the overall health of the patient. Some common surgical procedures used in the treatment of metastatic disease include resection, amputation, and palliative surgery. It should be noted that surgery for metastatic disease is usually only suggested for individuals who have severe, chronic symptoms or have not responded to other forms of treatment. It is important to get medical treatment for metastatic disease of the foot and ankle as soon as possible to prevent the cancer from spreading and to ensure the best possible outcomes. Early diagnosis and treatment can help to alleviate symptoms and improve the chances of a successful [49, 50].

3. Conclusion

The hindfoot is a complex and important part of the foot and ankle, and it is susceptible to a wide range of pathologies that can cause pain, swelling, and difficulty moving the foot and ankle. Some common hindfoot pathologies include posterior tibial tendinopathy, FHL tendinopathy, posterior ankle impingement syndrome, heel contusion, calcaneal and talar stress fractures, RA of the hindfoot, Paget disease of the hindfoot, osteomyelitis of the calcaneus, and metastatic disease of the foot and ankle.

Treatment for hindfoot pathologies may include a combination of medications, physical therapy, and lifestyle changes to reduce inflammation and manage pain. In severe cases, surgery may be necessary to repair or reconstruct damaged tissues or bones. It is important to seek medical treatment for hindfoot pathologies to prevent the condition from worsening and to maintain good function of the foot and ankle. Early diagnosis and treatment can help to alleviate symptoms and prevent further damage to the foot and ankle.

Conflict of interest

The authors declare no conflict of interest.

Author details

Elif Tuğçe Çil
Yeditepe University, İstanbul, Turkey

*Address all correspondence to: tugce.cill@gmail.com

References

[1] Gates LS, Arden NK, Hannan MT, Roddy E, Gill TK, Hill CL, et al. Prevalence of foot pain across an international consortium of population based cohorts. Arthritis Care and Research. 2019;**71**(5):661-670

[2] Perry J. Anatomy and biomechanics of the hindfoot. Clinical Orthopaedics. 1983;**177**:9-15

[3] Ghanem I, Massaad A, Assi A, Rizkallah M, Bizdikian AJ, Abiad RE, et al. Understanding the foot's functional anatomy in physiological and pathological conditions: The calcaneopedal unit concept. Journal of Children's Orthopaedics. 2019;**13**(2):134-146

[4] Choo YJ, Park CH, Chang MC. Rearfoot disorders and conservative treatment: A narrative review. Annals of Palliative Medicine. 2020;**9**(5):3546-3552

[5] Zimbler S, Craig C. Foot deformities. The Orthopedic Clinics of North America. 1976;**7**(29):331-339

[6] Maughan KL, Jackson J. Evaluation and Diagnosis of Common Causes of Hindfoot Pain in Adults—UpToDate. 2022. Available from: https://www.uptodate.com/contents/evaluation-and-diagnosis-of-common-causes-of-hindfoot-pain-in-adults

[7] Trojian T, Tucker AK. Plantar fasciitis. American Family Physician. 2019;**99**(12):744-750

[8] Lemont H, Ammirati KM, Usen N. Plantar fasciitis: A degenerative process (fasciosis) without inflammation. Journal of the American Podiatric Medical Association. 2003;**93**(3):234-237

[9] La Porta GA, La Fata PC. Pathologic conditions of the plantar fascia. Clinics in Podiatric Medicine and Surgery. 2005;**22**(1):1-9

[10] Buchanan BK, Kushner D. Plantar Fasciitis. In: StatPearls. Treasure Island (FL): StatPearls Publishing; 2022. Available from: http://www.ncbi.nlm.nih.gov/books/NBK431073

[11] Rhim HC, Kwon J, Park J, Stein JB, Tenforde AS. A systematic review of systematic reviews on the epidemiology, evaluation, and treatment of plantar fasciitis. Life. 2021;**11**(12):1287

[12] Çil ET, Şaylı U, Subaşı F. Outpatient vs home management protocol results for plantar fasciitis. Foot & Ankle International. 2019;**40**(11):1295-1303

[13] Drake C, Whittaker GA, Kaminski MR, Chen J, Keenan AM, Rathleff MS. Medical imaging for plantar heel pain: A systematic review and meta-analysis. Journal of Foot and Ankle Research. 2022;**15**(1):4

[14] Nelson SC. Tarsal Tunnel Syndrome. Clinics in Podiatric Medicine and Surgery. 2021;**38**(2):131-141

[15] McSweeney SC, Cichero M. Tarsal tunnel syndrome—A narrative literature review. Foot (Edinburgh, Scotland). 2015;**25**(4):244-250

[16] Grävare Silbernagel K, Malliaras P, de Vos R-J, Hanlon S, Molenaar M, Alfredson H, et al. ICON 2020—International scientific tendinopathy symposium consensus: A systematic review of outcome measures reported in clinical trials of Achilles tendinopathy. Sports Medicine. 2021;**52**(3):613-641

[17] van der Vlist AC, Breda SJ, Oei EHG, Verhaar JA, Jan de Vos R. Clinical risk factors for Achilles tendinopathy: A systematic review. British Journal of Sports Medicine. 2019;**53**(21):1352-1361

[18] Maffulli N, Sharma P, Luscombe KL. Achilles tendinopathy: Aetiology and management. Journal of the Royal Society of Medicine. 2004;**97**(10):472-476

[19] Kozlovskaia M, Vlahovich N, Ashton KJ, Hughes DC. Biomedical risk factors of Achilles tendinopathy in physically active people: A systematic review. Sports Medicine—Open. 2017;**3**(1):20

[20] Li H-Y, Hua Y-H. Achilles tendinopathy: Current concepts about the basic science and clinical treatments. BioMed Research International. 2016;**2016**:6492597

[21] Kang S, Thordarson DB, Charlton TP. Insertional Achilles tendinitis and Haglund's deformity. Foot & Ankle International. 2012;**33**(6):487-491

[22] Vaishya R, Agarwal AK, Azizi AT, Vijay V. Haglund's syndrome: A commonly seen mysterious condition. Cureus. 2016;**8**(10):e820

[23] Damiano J, Bouysset M. Douleurs de l'arrière-pied [Hindfoot pain]. Revue du praticien. 2010;**60**(3):353-360. French

[24] Arshad Z, Bhatia M. Current concepts in sinus tarsi syndrome: A scoping review. Foot and Ankle Surgery. 2021;**27**(6):615-621. DOI: 10.1016/j.fas.2020.08.013. Epub 2020 Sep 16

[25] Dozier TJ, Figueroa RT, Kalmar J. Sinus tarsi syndrome. Journal of the Louisiana State Medical Society. 2001;**153**(9):458-461

[26] André R, Laffitte E. Piezogenic pedal papules. Presse Médicale. 2019;**48**(1 Pt 1): 88. DOI: 10.1016/j.lpm.2018.09.018. Epub 2018 Dec 7

[27] Rocha Bde O, Fernandes JD, Prates FV. Piezogenic Pedal Papules. Anais Brasileiros de Dermatologia. 2015;**90**(6):928-929. DOI: 10.1590/abd1806-4841.20154884

[28] Kim JS, Amendola A, Barg A, Baumhauer J, Brodsky JW, Cushman DM, et al. Summary report of the Arthritis Foundation and the American Orthopaedic Foot & Ankle Society's symposium on targets for osteoarthritis research: Part 1: Epidemiology, pathophysiology, and current imaging approaches. Foot & Ankle Orthopaedics. 2022;**7**(4):24730114221127011. DOI: 10.1177/24730114221127011

[29] Andersen LB, Stauff MP, Juliano PJ. Combined subtalar and ankle arthritis. Foot and Ankle Clinics. 2007;**12**(1):57-73. DOI: 10.1016/j.fcl.2006.12.009

[30] Willegger M, Hirtler L, Schwarz GM, Windhager RH, Chiari C. Peronealsehnenpathologien: Von der diagnose bis zur Behandlung [Peroneal tendon pathologies: From the diagnosis to treatment]. Orthopade. 2021;**50**(7):589-604. DOI: 10.1007/s00132-021-04116-6. German. Epub 2021 Jun 23

[31] Roster B, Michelier P, Giza E. Peroneal tendon disorders. Clinics in Sports Medicine. 2015;**34**(4):625-641. DOI: 10.1016/j.csm.2015.06.003. Epub 2015 Jul 31

[32] Ling SK, Lui TH. Posterior tibial tendon dysfunction: An overview. The Open Orthopaedics Journal. 2017;**11**:714-723. DOI: 10.2174/1874325001711010714

[33] Simpson MR, Howard TM. Tendinopathies of the foot and ankle.

American Family Physician. 2009;**80**(10): 1107-1114

[34] Michelson J, Dunn L. Tenosynovitis of the flexor hallucis longus: A clinical study of the spectrum of presentation and treatment. Foot & Ankle International. 2005;**26**(4):291-303. DOI: 10.1177/107110070502600405

[35] Ishibashi MA, Doyle MD, Krcal CE Jr. Posterior Ankle Impingement Syndrome. Clinics in Podiatric Medicine and Surgery. 2023;**40**(1):209-222. DOI: 10.1016/j.cpm.2022.07.014. Epub 2022 Sep 28

[36] Nikolopoulos D, Safos G, Moustakas K, Sergides N, Safos P, Siderakis A, et al. Endoscopic treatment of posterior ankle impingement secondary to Os trigonum in recreational athletes. Foot & Ankle Orthopaedics. 2020;**5**(3):2473011420945330

[37] Bojanić I, Janjić T, Dimnjaković D, Križan S, Smoljanović T. Stražnji sindrom sraza gležnja [Posterior ankle impingement syndrome]. Lijec Vjesn. 2015;**137**(3-4):109-115. Croatian

[38] Conklin RJ. Common cutaneous disorders in athletes. Sports Medicine. 1990;**9**(2):100-119. DOI: 10.2165/00007256-199009020-00004

[39] Perry DR, O'Toole ED. Stress fracture of the talar neck and distal calcaneus. Journal of the American Podiatry Association. 1981;**71**(11):637-638. DOI: 10.7547/87507315-71-11-637

[40] Cimino WG, O'Malley MJ. Rheumatoid arthritis of the ankle and hindfoot. Rheumatic Diseases Clinics of North America. 1998;**24**(1):157-172. DOI: 10.1016/s0889-857x(05)70383-5

[41] Aronow MS, Hakim-Zargar M. Management of hindfoot disease in rheumatoid arthritis. Foot and Ankle Clinics. 2007;**12**(3):455-474, vi. DOI: 10.1016/j.fcl.2007.05.003

[42] Kravets I. Paget's disease of bone: Diagnosis and treatment. The American Journal of Medicine. 2018;**131**(11):1298-1303. DOI: 10.1016/j.amjmed.2018.04.028. Epub 2018 May 10

[43] Torre A, De Monti M. Osteomyelitis of the calcaneus with pathologic fracture. The Journal of Foot and Ankle Surgery. 2020;**59**(3):641. DOI: 10.1053/j.jfas.2019.09.022

[44] Chen K, Balloch R. Management of calcaneal osteomyelitis. Clinics in Podiatric Medicine and Surgery. 2010;**27**(3):417-429. DOI: 10.1016/j.cpm.2010.04.003

[45] Rees DC, Williams TN, Gladwin MT. Sickle-cell disease. Lancet. 2010;**376**(9757):2018-2031. DOI: 10.1016/S0140-6736(10)61029-X. Epub 2010 Dec 3

[46] Meier ER. Treatment options for sickle cell disease. Pediatric Clinics of North America. 2018;**65**(3):427-443. DOI: 10.1016/j.pcl.2018.01.005

[47] Dalbeth N, Gosling AL, Gaffo A, Abhishek A. Gout. Lancet. 2021;**397**(10287):1843-1855. DOI: 10.1016/S0140-6736(21)00569-9. Epub 2021 Mar 30. Erratum in: Lancet. 2021;397(10287):1808

[48] Bernal JA, García-Campos J, Marco-LLedó J, Andrés M. Gouty involvement of foot and ankle: Beyond flares. Reumatología Clínica (English Edition). 2021;**17**(2):106-112. DOI: 10.1016/j.reuma.2019.12.003. English, Spanish. Epub 2020 Feb 14

[49] Gall RJ, Sim FH, Pritchard DJ. Metastatic tumors to the bones of the

foot. Cancer. 1976;**37**(3): 1492-1495. DOI: 10.1002/1097-0142(197603)37:3<1492:: aid-cncr2820370335>3.0.co;2-q

[50] Wu KK, Guise ER. Metastatic tumors of the foot. Southern Medical Journal. 1978;**71**(7):807-808, 812. DOI: 10.1097/00007611-197807000-00021

Section 5

Achille Tendon Rupture

Chapter 6

Functional Rehabilitation after Achilles Tendon Rupture

Andrej Čretnik

Abstract

Optimal treatment of an acute Achilles tendon rupture remains controversial. There's but a clear tendency that either treated conservatively or operatively, patients should start as soon as possible with early functional rehabilitation. It should include an early range of motion exercises and controlled weightbearing protocol with the support of crutches. Softcast brace is a simple, effective, removable, individually adapted, and well-tolerated orthosis, that can be easily made, if necessary, replaced or changed, and safely used during the healing process and if necessary, in the further rehabilitation period. Proposed rehabilitation protocol with the use of a softcast brace can be used either in conservatively or operatively treated patients, with comparable results in terms of complication rate (re-ruptures, thromboembolic events, sural neuritis) and long-term clinical (ROM, length of tendon) and functional results (return to pre-injured activities).

Keywords: achilles tendon, rupture, functional rehabilitation, softcast brace, ROM exercises

1. Introduction

Controversy regarding the optimal treatment of an acute complete Achilles tendon rupture (ATR) remains despite great interest and several articles in the last decades. Treatment can be broadly classified into conservative management with cast immobilization or functional bracing [1–6] and operative management with open repair (with or without augmentation) [1–3, 5–7], or minimally invasive procedures with closed percutaneous repair [8–11], or semi-open techniques [12–15], with possible ultrasonography guidance [16, 17], or endoscopic control [18–20]. There are several postoperative rehabilitation protocols—traditionally, nonweightbearing, bellow knee cast immobilization is generally recommended for 6 to 8 weeks [1, 2, 6], that has changed in the last decades in mainly functional accelerated rehabilitation with functional bracing (including early ankle motion exercises and weightbearing) for the same period [2–5, 13, 16, 21–24].

Meta-analyses and quantitative reviews of the literature regarding the management of ATRs have shown that open-operative treatment was associated with a lower risk of re-rupture (pooled rate in the literature range from 1.4 to 5% [25–34]) than nonoperative management (pooled rate of re-rupture in the literature range from 2.4 to 13% [25–27, 29–35]. Systematic review and meta-analysis of 10 randomized controlled trials involving 944 patients and 19 observational studies, including 14,918 patients showed a significant reduction in re-ruptures after operative treatment (2.3%)

compared with nonoperative treatment (3.9%) (risk difference 1.6%; risk ratio 0.43, 95% confidence interval 0.31 to 0.60; $p < 0.001$; $I^2 = 22\%$), but with significantly higher complication rate in operative than nonoperative treatment (4.9 vs. 1.6%; risk difference 3.3%; risk ratio 2.76, 1.84 to 4.13; $p < 0.001$; $I^2 = 45\%$) [36]. The risk of complications could be possibly diminished by percutaneous repair (pooled rate of 26.1% in the open group vs. pooled rate of 8.3% in the percutaneous group) [30].

The concept of early dynamic functional rehabilitation has dramatically changed the results in a term of re-rupture rate, particularly in conservative treatment of ATR [4, 23, 37]. Meta-analysis of 10 randomized trials in 418 surgically treated patients and in 408 patients who underwent nonsurgical treatment showed that if functional rehabilitation with early range of motion (ROM) was employed, re-rupture rates were equal for surgical and nonsurgical patients (risk difference = 1.7%, p = 0.45), [37]. If such early ROM was not employed, the absolute risk reduction achieved by surgery was 8.8% (p = 0.001 in favor of surgery) [37]. Similar findings were also found in the largest systematic review and meta-analysis, with no statistically significant difference in re-rupture rate between operative and nonoperative treatment in studies that used accelerated functional rehabilitation (risk ratio 0.60, 0.26 to 1.37; p = 0.23; $I^2 = 0\%$) [36]. The beneficial impact of early dynamic functional rehabilitation has been proven only by both, early weightbearing and ankle motion exercises [38].

2. Functional rehabilitation after Achilles tendon rupture

2.1 Immobilization and orthoses

According to the literature, there are several options available for functional treatment after ATR. Generally, they can be divided into different, mainly individually (custom) made splints, (semi)casts or orthoses from cast or different plastic materials and various special shoes, boots, or walkers (**Figures 1** and **2**) and prefabricated braces and orthoses, manufactured by different medical companies.

As functional rehabilitation should consist of early weightbearing and range of motion (ROM) exercises, there are various solutions proposed for that among previously listed types of immobilization. In rigid types of semi-casts, at least two different casts should be made—first in the plantar flexion of foot for about 25 to 30 degrees and after 3 weeks in the neutral position. In the last decades, plantar flexion is recommended to be changed every second week— every time for about 10 degrees, so at the end of a period of 6-weeks of immobilization, a neutral position of the foot could be achieved, with gradually increased tension to the injured AT, what seems to bring a beneficial effect to the strength and therefore to lower re-rupture rate [23, 37, 39, 40]. In orthoses, made from softcast or soft-plastic materials, reduction of the plantar flexion of the foot to a neutral position can be gradually achieved with the softening of the orthosis with the increased weightbearing and thus providing all the time the increase of the tension to the injured AT, with the same possibly beneficial effect of reducing the re-rupture rate [39].

In various special shoes, boots, or walkers' plantar flexion can be achieved with the added special heel lifts that can be diminished every week by 0.5 cm or every 2 weeks for 1 cm (**Figure 2**). Some of these special boots or walkers have a hinge at the level of tibiotalar joint, which can be locked in a desired position or can restrict plantar flexion at the beginning from 30 to 50 degrees and then gradually every week more, toward 0 to 50 degrees (**Figure 3**). With the addition of heel lift, early controlled weightbearing can be achieved, too.

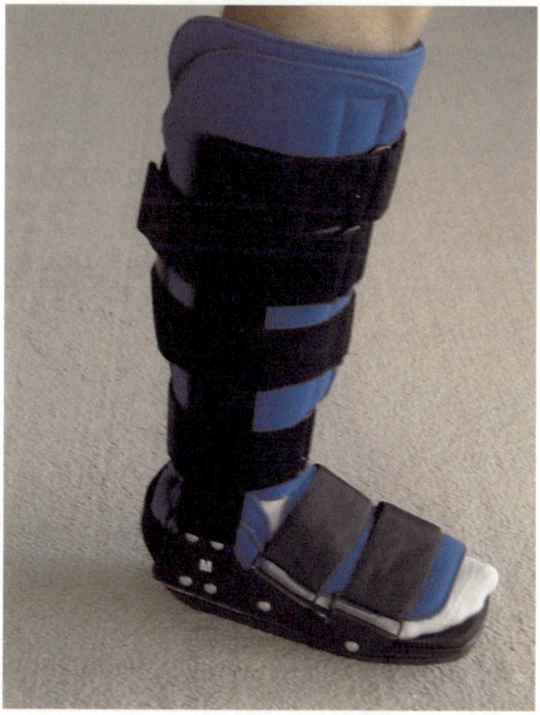

Figure 1.
Walker.

2.2 Softcast functional orthosis

Simple, but effective and individually adjusted orthosis is presented on **Figures 4–6**. It can be used in conservative as well as in operative treatment, whether in an open or minimally invasive way. Generally, it's applied with the foot at 25 degrees PF. Long stockinette (3 M, St. Paul, MN) (**Figure 4**) is dorsally covered with the splint, made of several (5) folded layers of Softcast (3 M, St. Paul, MN) (**Figure 5**). The splint is fixed with a folded stockinette or a simple (additional) bandage, which enables patients to perform PF and prevents dorsiflexion (DF) (**Figure 6**).

2.3 Rehabilitation protocol

Patients are immediately allowed to walk with crutches in a toe-touch technique. In the next 2 to 3 days, they can carefully increase weightbearing (WB) to 5 kg and then every week for an additional 5 kg, reaching so 15 kg of weightbearing within first 3 weeks (about 25% of body-weight (BW)). They should be immediately encouraged also to perform ROM exercises, as much as their immobilization allows (**Figure 6**).

After a week, patients are allowed to take off and on brace during the day and to perform careful PF and DF between 25 and 50 degrees in a seating position (in water without orthosis). The useful tip should be recommended to the patients, to perform ROM exercises and weightbearing only until the pain is felt.

After 2 weeks, patients should be encouraged to continue with increasing weightbearing for 5 kg every week, continuously with gradation until pain is felt.

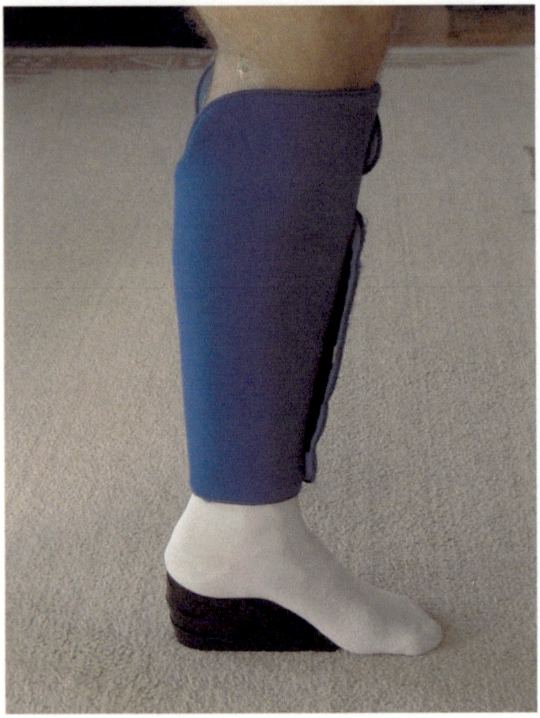

Figure 2.
Heel support.

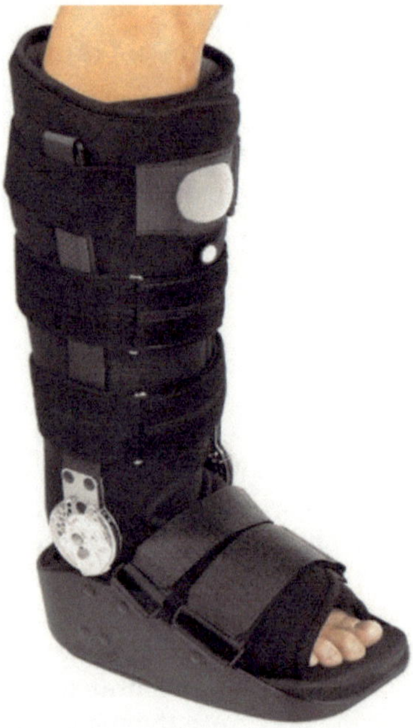

Figure 3.
Walker with the locking mechanism.

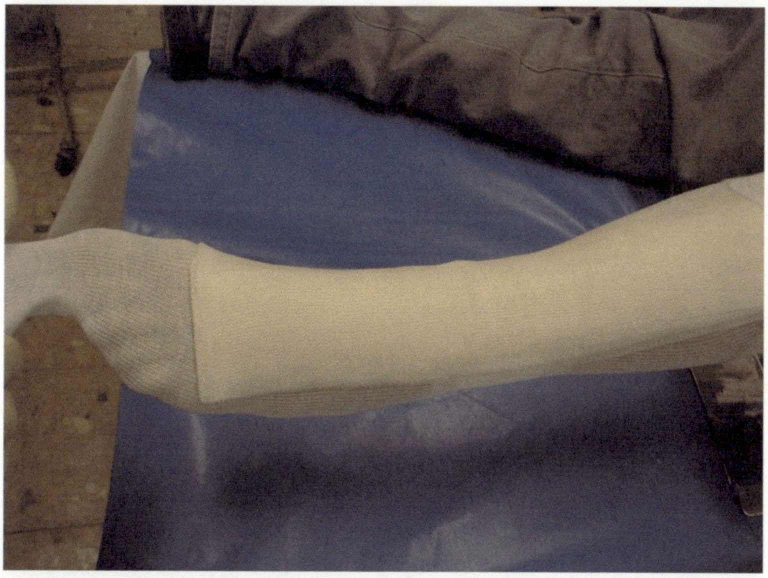

Figure 4.
Softcast functional orthosis—Preparation with stockinette).

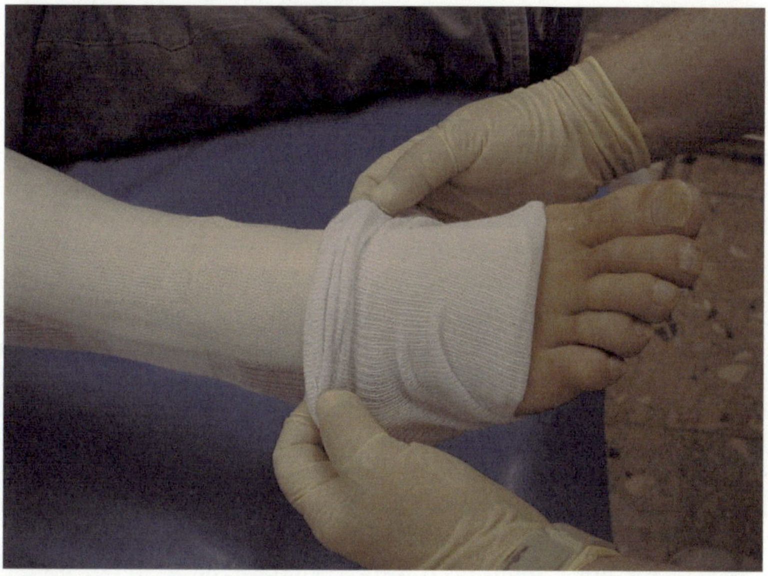

Figure 5.
Softcast functional orthosis–folding stockinette.

After 4 week, they can start with weightbearing as much as tolerated and if they have no pain, they can start to walk even without crutches but should be very cautious if walking on a wet or slippery floor. Softcast (functional) immobilization routinely softens with weightbearing, so there is no need to exchange this type of immobilization to achieve a neutral position of the foot. On the other hand, this is also a way of controlling patients about weightbearing.

Bilateral seated ROM exercises, with a progressive increase of dorsiflexion and force (pain) controlled pushing knee by hands (ankle down until pain is felt), should

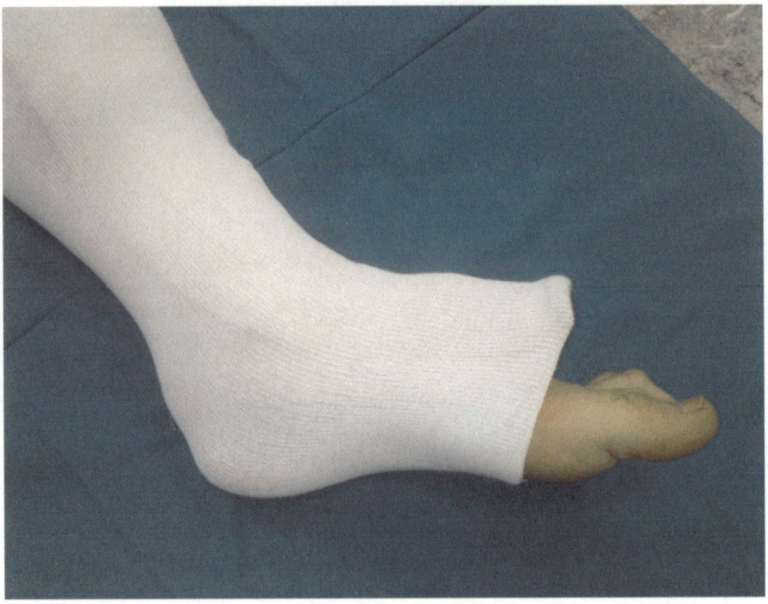

Figure 6.
ROM exercises—Plantar flexion in orthosis.

be encouraged according to the protocol in **Table 1** to reach a neutral position of the foot within 6 weeks (**Figures 6** and 7).

After 6 weeks, immobilization can be removed, and patients should start with the rehabilitation protocol (learned and controlled by physiotherapists). They may walk without crutches, with progressively increasing weightbearing (till tolerable pain). ROM exercises with increasing DF above the neutral position should also be performed carefully—it's recommended till 8 weeks in the sitting position and if possible, in the water.

Special attention should be given to incorrect gait patterns. Generally, no additional heel pad or cushion is recommended. Patients should be encouraged to perform as much as possible exercises in the whirlpool, where full weightbearing is allowed.

Careful stretching exercises and controlled squats with a lifted heel could be started after 8 weeks with careful increasing of the load (until pain is felt). Full active dorsiflexion is expected to be reached after 4 months. Raising on toes or heels with the operated leg only is generally allowed 12 weeks after the operation. Sports activities should be carefully started and individually adjusted after 3 months, with recommended full loading 6 months after the operation. Steps in rehabilitation are summarized in **Table 1**.

Proposed early dynamic functional rehabilitation with softcast orthosis can be successfully implemented with conservative as well as other open, semi-open, or closed percutaneous methods, too, as there are no contraindications for this type of treatment.

Long-term results with the use of proposed early dynamic functional rehabilitation, together with the closed percutaneous repair under local anesthesia, can be compared to other methods of ATR in terms of complication rate (re-ruptures, thromboembolic events, sural neuritis, etc.) and long term clinical (ROM, length of tendon) and functional results (strength and return to pre-injured activities) [16, 39].

2.4 Functional rehabilitation program (never exceed pain)

0 to 1 week		
Immobilization, Plantar flexion 25°	Crutches, Toe-touch/5 kg weightbearing (WB)	Gait control
1 to 2 weeks		
Immobilization, Plantar flexion 20°	Crutches, 5–10 kg WB, bathing	Seated ROM exercises
2 to 3 weeks		
Immobilization, Plantar flexion 15°	Crutches, 10–15 kg WB (20%BW)	Seated/pushing exercises
3 to 4 weeks		
Immobilization, Plantar flexion 10°	Crutches, 15–20 kg WB (30%BW)	Seated/pushing exercises
4 to 5 weeks		
Immobilization, Plantar flexion 5°	Crutches*, 20–25 kg WB (40%BW) (as tolerated)	Seated/pushing exercises
5 to 6 weeks		
Immobilization, Plantar flexion 0°	Crutches*, 25–30 kg WB (50%BW) (as tolerated)	Seated/pushing exercises
6 to 8 weeks – starting with physiotherapy		
No immobilization, Dorsiflexion+5°	No crutches, walking with weightbearing	Careful swimming
Control swelling (Ultrasonography, laser, negative pressure ...), massage Gait control / no limping, careful weightbearing on slippery surfaces Pain controlled strength and endurance exercises (cycling, walking on treadmill, hydrotherapy)		
8 to 10 weeks		
Active dorsiflexion +10°	Walking with normal weightbearing	Bilateral raising on toes
Graduated resistance exercises (pain controlled) (skipping with leaning on hands, (light) cycling, treadmill ...) Careful stretching, friction massage ... Proprioception exercises (controlled), NO jumping, sprinting, sudden loading, etc.		
10 to 12 weeks		
Active dorsiflexion +15°	Walking with full weightbearing	Gradual raising with OP leg
Progress of resistance exercises (pain controlled), (careful start—light sports activities, warming/stretching ...)		
12 to 16 weeks		
Active dorsiflexion +20°	Fast walking, careful jogging, running	Raising on toes with OP leg
Pain controlled progress of resistance and endurance exercises, sports activities, eccentric exercises (retrain strength, power, dynamic weightbearing exercises ...) (individually adapted according to progress)		
After 16 weeks		
Gradual return to sports activities—individually adapted—if no pain, increasing activities like running, jumping, sprinting, sudden loading, etc.		
After 6 months		
Generally, return to all sports activities (take care about tendinopathy /warming, stretching, strengthening)		

Table 1.
Rehabilitation protocol in steps.

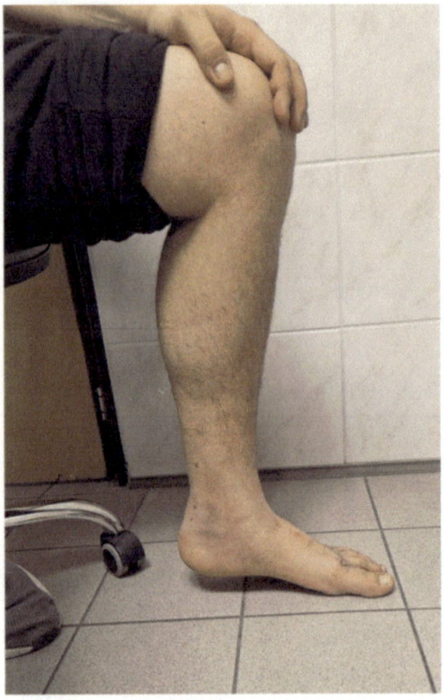

Figure 7.
Pushing knee in a seated position—Increasing dorsiflexion of ankle.

3. Discussion

Restoration of the length and tension of the ruptured AT with the return to preinjury activities with as less complications as possible should be the goals of the treatment of ATR. As in complete ATR, there always come to retraction of the triceps muscle. Consequently, a gap (elongated tendon) remains between torn ends, which heals in conservative treatment with fibrous tissue [16, 39]. Due to biomechanical characteristics of the musculotendinous complex, elongation of less than 0.5 cm seems not to affect AT function in basic daily activities but might be important in high-caliber athletes [16, 39, 41–43]. Open surgical repair enables restoration of the original length, together with tendon augmentation, but poses a higher risk for complications [5, 7, 16]. Percutaneous repair, particularly semi-open with the possible control of the length (Achillon® system (Integra Life Sciences Corporation, Plainsboro, NJ), PARS™ system (Arthrex, Naples, FL), Achilles midsubstance Speed Bridge repair variation (Arthrex, Naples, FL) [12–15] or closed percutaneous repair with ultrasonographical control [10, 16, 17, 39], seems to bridge the gap, particularly with reducing the overall number of complications.

The results of studies support a beneficial effect of early functional rehabilitation with all types of ATR treatment. Wu et al. found in their systematic review and network meta-analysis of 2060 patients in 29 randomized controlled trials 7.41% of overall complication rates in the group of open surgery and accelerated rehabilitation in comparison to 8.47% in the group of minimally invasive surgery and accelerated rehabilitation, 12.09% in nonsurgery group and accelerated rehabilitation and 13.97% in nonsurgery group and early immobilization [44].

It has to be stressed that weightbearing and early ROM exercises before the healing of an ATR could have some detrimental effects, too. Eliasson et al. found in their study that ruptured AT elongates for 6 months after surgical repair regardless of early or late weightbearing in combination with ankle mobilization [45]. Kangas et al. and Mortensen et al. also showed separation of the tendon ends during the postoperative period and Lee et al. and Clanton et al. warned in their studies about gapping in cycling loading, which might cause tendon elongation [22, 46–48]. Weakness of plantar flexion strength, together with a deficit in heel-rise test in patients with ATR could therefore be explained with tendon elongation [49, 50].

Strength of the tendon repair with the resistance to elongation during loading could possibly have an impact on the final results, so generally with any type of operative treatment, the strongest repair should be considered [39].

Probably the simplest way to achieve the goals of accelerated rehabilitation (early weightbearing with early ROM exercises), could be the adjustment of all activities to the proportion of pain. Proposed kg of weightbearing in weekly intervals should probably serve only as a sort of general recommendation, which should be individually adjusted (according to body weight), as it has no sense to compare 5 kg of weightbearing in 100 kg body-weight man, with a lady of 50 kg body-weight.

Functional treatment with early ankle motion and early weightbearing might have an impact on the negative effect of immobilization and thus risk for deep venous thrombosis (DVT) and venous thromboembolism (VTE) [39]. There is but no clear consensus about the incidence of VTE and prophylaxis in patients after ATR and it seems that patient-specific risk factors for VTE should be assessed individually [51–54]. The American College of Chest Physicians' (ACCP) review recommends against chemical prophylaxis in lower leg injuries requiring immobilization [53]. Functional treatment and early ankle motion could support this decision easier.

4. Conclusion

Controversy regarding optimal treatment after ATR remains. There's but clear tendency that either treated conservatively or operatively, patients should start as soon as possible with early functional rehabilitation.

Softcast brace is a simple, cheap, effective, removable, individually adapted, and well-tolerated orthosis, that can be easily made and safely used, together with the use of crutches, during the healing and rehabilitation process of the ruptured AT.

Long-term results support the choice of the proposed functional method for the patients with acute, complete ATR as the method that brings promising end functional results, with a low rate of complications.

Author details

Andrej Čretnik
Department of Traumatology, University Clinical Center, Maribor, Slovenia

*Address all correspondence to: andrej.cretnik@guest.arnes.si

References

[1] Cetti R, Christensen SE, Ejsted R. Operative versus nonoperative treatment of Achilles tendon rupture. The American Journal of Sports Medicine. 1993;**21**:791-799

[2] Nilsson-Helander K, Silbernagel KG, Thomeé R, Faxén E, Olsson N, Eriksson BI, et al. Acute Achilles tendon rupture: A randomized, controlled study comparing surgical and nonsurgical treatments using validated outcome measures. The American Journal of Sports Medicine. 2010;**38**:2186-2193

[3] Willits K, Amendola A, Bryant D, Mohtadi NG, Giffin JR, Fowler P, et al. Operative versus nonoperative treatment of acute Achilles tendon ruptures: A multicenter randomized trial using accelerated functional rehabilitation. Journal of Bone and Joint Surgery-American. 2010;**92**(17): 2767-2775

[4] Wallace RGH, Heyes GJ, Michael ALR. The non-operative functional management of patients with a rupture of the tendo Achillis leads to low rates of rerupture. The Journal of Bone and Joint Surgery. British. 2011;**93**: 1362-1366

[5] Olsson N, Silbernagel KG, Eriksson BI, Sansone M, Brorsson A, Nilsson-Hellander K, et al. Stable surgical repair with accelerated rehabilitation versus nonsurgical treatment for acute Achilles tendon ruptures: A randomized controlled study. The American Journal of Sports Medicine. 2013;**41**:2867-2876

[6] Lantto I, Heikkinen J, Flinkkila T, Ohtonen P, Siira P, Laine V, et al. A prospective randomized trial comparing surgical and nonsurgical treatments of acute Achilles tendon ruptures. The American Journal of Sports Medicine. 2016;**44**:2406-2414

[7] Heikkinen J, Lantto I, Flinkkila T, Ohtonen P, Pajala A, Siira P, et al. Augmented compared with nonaugmented surgical repair after total Achilles rupture: Results of a prospective randomized trial with thirteen or more years of follow-up. Journal of Bone and Joint Surgery-American. 2016;**98**:85-92

[8] Ma GWC, Griffith TG. Percutaneous repair of acute closed ruptured Achilles tendon: A new technique. Clinical Orthopaedics. 1977;**128**:247-255

[9] Kosanović M, Čretnik A, Batišta M. Subcutaneous suturing of the ruptured Achilles tendon under local anesthesia. Archives of Orthopaedic and Trauma Surgery. 1994;**113**:177-179

[10] Čretnik A, Smrkolj V, Kosanović M. Percutaneous suturing of the ruptured Achilles tendon under local anesthesia. The Journal of Foot and Ankle Surgery. 2004;**43**(2):72-81

[11] Amlang MH, Christiani P, Heinz P, Zwipp H. The percutaneous suture of the Achilles tendon with the Dresden instrument. Operative Orthopädie und Traumatologie. 2006;**18**(4): 287-299

[12] Kakiuchi M. A combined open and percutaneous technique for repair of tendon Achillis. Comparison with open repair. Journal of Bone & Joint Surgery. 1995;**77B**:60-63

[13] Buchgraber A, Pässler HH. Percutaneous repair of Achilles tendon rupture. Immobilization versus functional postoperative treatment. Clinical Orthopaedics. 1997;**341**:113-122

[14] Assal M, Jung M, Stern R, Rippstein P, Delmi M, Hoffmeyer P. Limited open repair of Achilles tendon ruptures. A technique with a new instrument and findings of a prospective multicenter study. Journal of Bone & Joint Surgery. 2002;**84A**:161-170

[15] Hsu AR, Jones CP, Cohen BE, Davis WH, Ellington JK, Anderson RB. Clinical outcomes and complications of percutaneous Achilles repair system versus open technique for acute Achilles tendon rupture. Foot & Ankle International. 2015;**36**:1279-1286

[16] Čretnik A, Smrkolj V, Kosanović M. Percutaneous versus open repair of the ruptured Achilles tendon. A comparative study. The American Journal of Sports Medicine. 2005;**33**:1369-1379

[17] Soubeyrand M, Serra-Tosio G, Campagna R, Molina V, Sitbon P, Biau DJ. Intraoperative ultrasonography during percutaneous Achilles tendon repair. Foot and Ankle International. 2010;**31**(12):1069-1074

[18] Halasi T, Tallay A, Berkes I. Percutaneous Achilles tendon repair with and without endoscopic control. Knee Surgery, Sports Traumatology, Arthroscopy. 2003;**11**:409-414

[19] Tang KL, Therman H, Dai G, Chen GX, Guo L, Yang L. Arthroscopically assisted percutaneous repair of fresh closed Achilles tendon rupture by Kessler's suture. The American Journal of Sports Medicine. 2007;**35**:589-596

[20] Doral MN, Bozkurt M, Turhan E, Ayvaz M, Atay OA, Uzumcugil A, et al. Percutaneous suturing of the ruptured Achilles tendon using endoscopic control. Archives of Orthopaedic and Trauma Surgery. 2009;**129**: 1093-1101

[21] McComis GP, Nawoczenski DA, DeHaven KE. Functional bracing for rupture of the Achilles tendon. Clinical results and analysis of ground-reaction forces and temporal data. Journal of Bone & Joint Surgery. 1997;**79A**:1799-1808

[22] Mortensen HM, Skov O, Jensen PE. Early motion of the ankle after operative treatment of a rupture of the Achilles tendon. A prospective, randomized clinical and radiographic study. The Journal of Bone and Joint Surgery American. 1999;**81**:983-990

[23] Twaddle BC, Poon P. Early motion for Achilles tendon ruptures: Is surgery important? A randomized prospective study. The American Journal of Sports Medicine. 2007;**35**(12):2033-2038

[24] Lantto I, Heikkinen J, Flinkkila T, Ohtonen P, Kangas J, Siira P, et al. Early functional treatment versus cast immobilization in tension after achilles rupture repair: Results of a prospective randomized trial with 10 or more years of follow-up. The American Journal of Sports Medicine. 2015;**43**:2302-2309

[25] Wong J, Barrass V, Maffulli N. Quantitative review of operative and nonoperative management of Achilles tendon ruptures. The American Journal of Sports Medicine. 2002;**30**:565-575

[26] Wang D, Sandlin MI, Cohen JR, Lord EL, Petrigliano FA, Nelson F, et al. Operative versus nonoperative treatment of acute Achilles tendon rupture: An analysis of 12,570 patients in a large healthcare database. Foot and Ankle Surgery. 2017;**21**:250-253

[27] Kocher MS, Bishop J, Marshall R, Briggs KK, Hawkins RJ. Operative versus nonoperative management of acute achilles tendon rupture. Expected-value decision analysis. The American Journal of Sports Medicine. 2002;**30**:783-790

[28] Attia AK, Mahmoud K, d'Hooghe P, Bariteau J, Labib SA, Myerson MS. Outcomes and complications of open versus minimally invasive repair of acute Achilles tendon ruptures. A systematic review and meta-analysis of randomized controlled trials. The American Journal of Sports Medicine. 2021;**49**:1-12. DOI: 10.1177/03635465211053619

[29] Bhandari M, Guyatt GH, Siddiqui F, Morrow F, Busse J, Leighton RK, et al. Treatment of acute Achilles tendon ruptures: A systematic overview and meta-analysis. Clinical Orthopaedics and Related Research. 2002;**400**: 190-200

[30] Khan RJ, Fick D, Keogh A, Crawford J, Brammar T, Parker M. Treatment of acute Achilles tendon ruptures: A meta-analysis of randomized, controlled trials. The Journal of Bone and Joint Surgery American. 2005;**87**:2202-2210

[31] Wilkins R, Bisson LJ. Operative versus nonoperative management of acute Achilles tendon ruptures: A quantitative systematic review of randomized controlled trials. The American Journal of Sports Medicine. 2012;**40**:2154-2160

[32] Deng S, Sun Z, Zhang C, Chen G, Li J. Surgical treatment versus conservative management for acute Achilles tendon rupture: A systematic review and meta-analysis of randomized controlled trials. The Journal of Foot and Ankle Surgery. 2017;**56**: 1236-1243

[33] van der Eng DM, Schepers T, Goslings JC, Schep NW. Rerupture rate after early weightbearing in operative versus conservative treatment of Achilles tendon ruptures: A meta-analysis. The Journal of Foot and Ankle Surgery. 2013;**52**:622-628

[34] Jones MP, Khan RJ, Carey Smith RL. Surgical interventions for treating acute achilles tendon rupture: Key findings from a recent Cochrane review. The Journal of Bone and Joint Surgery American. 2012;**94**:e88

[35] Khan RJ, Carey Smith RL. Surgical interventions for treating acute Achilles tendon ruptures. The Cochrane Database of Systematic Reviews. 2010;**9**: CD003674

[36] Ochen Y, Beks RB, van Heijl M, Hietbrink F, Leenen LPH, van der Velde D, et al. Operative treatment versus nonoperative treatment of Achilles tendon ruptures: Systematic review and meta-analysis. BMJ. 2019; **364**:k5120

[37] Soroceanu A, Sidhwa F, Aarabi S, Kaufman A, Glazebrook M. Surgical versus nonsurgical treatment of acute Achilles tendon rupture: A meta-analysis of randomized trials. The Journal of Bone and Joint Surgery American. 2012;**94**: 2136-2143

[38] Huang J, Wang C, Ma X, Wang X, Zhang C, Chen L. Rehabilitation regimen after surgical treatment of acute Achilles tendon ruptures: A systematic review with meta-analysis. The American Journal of Sports Medicine. 2015;**43**: 1008-1016

[39] Čretnik A, Kosanović M, Košir R. Long-term results with the use of modified percutaneous repair of the ruptured Achilles tendon under local anaesthesia: (15-year analysis with 270 cases). The Journal of Foot and Ankle Surgery. 2019;**58**:828-836

[40] Costa MI, Achten J, Dutton S, Lamb SE, Ollivere B, Maredza M, et al. Plaster cast versus functional brace for non-surgical treatment of Achilles tendon rupture (UKSTAR): A

multicentre randomised controlled trial and economic evaluation. Lancet. 2020; **395**:441-448

[41] Kangas JA, Pajala A, Siira P, Hamalainen M, Leppilahti J. Early functional treatment versus early immobilization in tension of the musculotendinous unit after Achilles rupture repair: A prospective randomized, clinical study. The Journal of Trauma. 2003;**54**:1171-1180

[42] Zellers JA, Carmont MR, Silbernagel KG. Return to play post-Achilles tendon rupture: A systematic review and meta-analysis of rate and measures of return to play. British Journal of Sports Medicine. 2016;**50**: 1325-1332

[43] Trofa DP, Miller JC, Jang ES, Woode DR, Greisberg JK, Vosseller JT. Professional Athletes' return to play and performance after operative repair of an Achilles tendon rupture. The American Journal of Sports Medicine. 2017;**45**: 2864-2871

[44] Wu Y, Mu Y, Yin L, Wang Z, Liu W, Wan H. Complications in the management of acute Achilles tendon rupture. A systematic review and network meta-analysis of 2060 patients. The American Journal of Sports Medicine. 2019;**40**:2154-2160

[45] Eliasson PT, Agergaard A, Couppe C, Svensson R, Hoeffner R, Warming S, et al. The ruptured Achilles tendon elongates for 6 months after surgical repair regardless of early or late weightbearing in combination with ankle mobilization: A randomized clinical trial. The American Journal of Sports Medicine. 2018;**46**:2492-2502

[46] Kangas J, Pajala A, Ohtonen P, Leppilahti J. Achilles tendon elongation after rupture repair: A randomized comparison of 2 postoperative regimens. The American Journal of Sports Medicine. 2007;**35**:59-64

[47] Lee SJ, Sileo MJ, Kremenic IJ, Orishimo K, Ben-Avi S, Nicholas SJ, et al. Cyclic loading of 3 Achilles tendon repairs simulating early postoperative forces. The American Journal of Sports Medicine. 2009;**37**:786-790

[48] Clanton TO, Haytmanek CT, Williams BT, Civitaresse DM, Turnbull TL, Massey MB, et al. A biomechanical comparison of an open repair and 3 minimally invasive percutaneous Achilles tendon repairs during a simulated progressive rehabilitation protocol. The American Journal of Sports Medicine. 2015;**43**: 1957-1964

[49] Silbernagel KG, Steele R, Manal K. Deficits in heel-rise height and Achilles tendon elongation occur in patients recovering from an Achilles tendon rupture. The American Journal of Sports Medicine. 2012;**40**:1564-1571

[50] Rosso C, Vavken P, Polzer C, Buckland DM, Studler U, Weisskopf L, et al. Long-term outcomes of muscle volume and Achilles tendon length after Achilles tendon ruptures. Knee Surgery, Sports Traumatology, Arthroscopy. 2013;**21**:1369-1377

[51] Aufwerber S, Heijne A, Edman G, Silbernagel KG, Ackermann PW. Early mobilization does not reduce the risk of deep venous thrombosis after Achilles tendon rupture: A randomized controlled trial. Knee Surgery, Sports Traumatology, Arthroscopy. 2020;**28**: 312-319

[52] Calder JDF, Freeman R, Domeij-Arverud E, van Dijk CN, Ackermannn PW. Meta-analysis and suggested guidelines for prevention of

venous thromboembolism (VTE) in foot and ankle surgery. Knee Surgery, Sports Traumatology, Arthroscopy. 2016;**24**: 1409-1420

[53] Falck-Ytter Y, Francis CW, Johanson NA, Curley C, Dahl OE, Schulman S, et al. Prevention of VTE in orthopedic surgery patients: Antithrombotic therapy and prevention of thrombosis, 9th ed: American College of Chest Physicians evidence-based clinical practice guidelines. Chest. 2012; **141**(2 Suppl):278S-325S

[54] Patel A, Ogawa B, Charlton T, Thordarson D. Incidence of deep vein thrombosis and pulmonary embolism after Achilles tendon rupture. Clinical Orthopaedics and Related Research. 2012;**470**:270-274